The Reproductive System at a Glance

This title is also available as an e-book.
For more details, please see
www.wiley.com/buy/9781118607039
or scan this QR code:

The Reproductive System at a Glance

Fourth Edition

Linda J. Heffner

PhD, MD
Professor of Obstetrics and Gynecology
Professor of Physiology and Biophysics
Boston University School of Medicine
Boston, MA
USA

Danny J. Schust

MD
David G. Hall Professor of Obstetrics and Gynecology
University Missouri School of Medicine
Chief, Division of Reproductive Endocrinology and Fertility
Department of Obstetrics, Gynecology and Women's Health
Missouri Women's and Children's Hospital
Columbia, MO
USA

WILEY Blackwell

This edition first published 2014 © 2014 by John Wiley & Sons, Ltd.
Third and Second editions published 2010; 2006 © 2010; 2006 by Linda J. Heffner and Danny J. Schust
First edition published 2001 © 2001 by John Wiley & Sons Ltd.

Registered office: John Wiley & Sons, Ltd, The Atrium, Southern Gate, Chichester, West Sussex, PO19
                       8SQ, UK

Editorial offices: 9600 Garsington Road, Oxford, OX4 2DQ, UK
                       The Atrium, Southern Gate, Chichester, West Sussex, PO19 8SQ, UK
                       111 River Street, Hoboken, NJ 07030-5774, USA

For details of our global editorial offices, for customer services and for information about how to apply
for permission to reuse the copyright material in this book please see our website at www.wiley.com/
wiley-blackwell

The right of the authors to be identified as the authors of this work has been asserted in accordance with
the UK Copyright, Designs and Patents Act 1988.

Library of Congress Cataloging-in-Publication Data

Heffner, Linda J., author.
  The reproductive system at a glance / Linda J. Heffner, Danny J. Schust. – Fourth edition.
      p. ; cm. – (At a glance series)
  Includes bibliographical references and index.
  ISBN 978-1-118-60703-9 (pbk. : alk. paper)
  I. Schust, Danny J., author. II. Title. III. Series: At a glance series (Oxford, England)
  [DNLM: 1. Reproduction–physiology. 2. Reproductive Physiological Processes. 3. Genital
Diseases, Female. 4. Genital Diseases, Male. 5. Pregnancy Complications. 6. Sexually Transmitted
Diseases. WQ 205]
  QP251
  612.6–dc23
                                2014000047

A catalogue record for this book is available from the British Library.

Wiley also publishes its books in a variety of electronic formats. Some content that appears in print may
not be available in electronic books.

Cover image: iStock/ © Ugurhan Betin
Cover design by Andy Meaden (Meaden Creative)

Set in 9/11.5 pt Times by Toppan Best-set Premedia Limited
Printed and bound in Malaysia by Vivar Printing Sdn Bhd

1 2014

Contents

Preface

Now in its fourth edition, *The Reproductive System at a Glance* is a comprehensive, easy-to-use collation of all the pertinent information on human reproductive processes and their diseases.

The most notable change between this edition and the last is the inclusion of an expanded supplementary material section. This includes multiple choice and short answer questions with detailed answers for each chapter. These questions are designed to help the student/reader determine if he or she has understood the important concepts. New material has been added to expand on normal maternal physiology in pregnancy and several new figures include pathology or radiologic images. All chapters and figures have been updated where new information is available.

The book remains divided into two parts. Part 1, which consists of 25 chapters, covers the normal human reproductive tract, continuing on through puberty with the resulting mature male and female anatomy and physiology and finally, procreation, pregnancy and menopause. Part 2, which consists of 23 chapters, covers the pathophysiology of anatomic, physiologic and psychologic disorders that interfere with normal reproductive function or health. Seven of these chapters are devoted to the more common malignancies that involve the reproductive organs.

Like its predecessor and the other books in this series, *The Reproductive System at a Glance* is written so that each topic is confined to a discrete vignette with appropriate illustrations or tables in a double page format. In Part 2, each topic also follows a standard format of a description of the disorder followed by its epidemiology, pathophysiology and, whenever it aids in understanding the disorder, a brief description of the commonly used treatments.

Revising a book, while easier than writing the original, remains a major undertaking to which many people contributed. We would like to thank Drs. Elizabeth Stier and David Wang for the helpful reviews on the chapters on human papillomavirus and cervical cancer, and male reproductive disorders, respectively. We would also like to thank the Obstetrics and Gynecology and Women's Health residents at the University of Missouri–Columbia for their invaluable help in creating the MCQ study guide questions for this text and Drs. A.J. Enciso, Taylor Hahn, Greg Blair and Megan Morman for help in fashioning MCQ answers and short answer questions and answers.

Finally, books never appear in print or on bookshelves without publishers. We would like to thank Elizabeth Johnston, Andrew Hallam and Karen Moore at Wiley Blackwell and also Jan East for assistance in producing this new edition. David Gardner was invaluable in revising old and drawing new figures.

Linda J. Heffner
Danny J. Schust
Boston and Columbia, 2013

Contributors

Gregory Blair, MD
Angel J. Enciso, MD
Taylor A. Hahn, MD
Megan M. Morman, MD

All at University of Missouri School of Medicine
Columbia, MO, USA

Table and figure acknowledgements

The following figures and tables have been redrawn from the originals and were used with permission of the publishers. Every effort has been made by the authors to contact all copyright holders to obtain their permission to reproduce copyright material. However, if any have been inadvertently overlooked, the publisher will be pleased to make the necessary arrangements at the earliest opportunity.

1 The pituitary gland and gonadotropins
Figure 1.1(a): Braunstein G (1989) Placental hormones, hormonal preparation for and control of parturition, and hormonal diagnosis of pregnancy. In: *Endocrinology* (ed. LJ deGroot), p.2045. Elsevier, Philadelphia.
Figure 1.1(b): Halvorsen LM, Chin WW (1999) Gonadotropic hormones: biosynthesis, secretion, receptors, and action. In: *Reproductive Endocrinology* (eds SSC Yen, RB Jaffe, RL Barbieri), p.92. Elsevier, Philadelphia.

2 Steroid hormone biosynthesis
Figure 2.2: Yeh J, Adashi EY (1999) The ovarian life cycle. In: *Reproductive Endocrinology* (eds SSC Yen, RB Jaffe, RL Barbieri), p.168. Elsevier, Philadelphia.

3 Steroid hormone mechanism of action and metabolism
Figure 3.1: O'Malley BW, Strott CA (1999) Steroid hormones: metabolism and mechanism of action. In: *Reproductive Endocrinology* (eds SSC Yen, RB Jaffe, RL Barbieri), p.124. Elsevier, Philadelphia.

4 Reproductive genetics
Figure 4.1: Morton CC, Miron P (1999) Cytogenetics. In: *Reproductive Endocrinology* (eds SSC Yen, RB Jaffe, RL Barbieri), p.337. Elsevier, Philadelphia.

5 Gonadal development in the embryo
Figure 5.1: Morton CC, Miron P (1999) Cytogenetics. Adapted from *Reproductive Endocrinology* (eds SSC Yen, RB Jaffe, RL Barbieri), p.337. Elsevier, Philadelphia.
Figure 5.2: Williams PL, Wendell – Smith CP, Treadgold S (1966) *Basic Human Embryology*, p.76. Lippincott Williams & Wilkins, Baltimore.

6 Phenotypic sex differentiation
Figure 6.1: Blainsky BI (1970) *An Introduction to Embryology*, 3rd edn, p.497. Elsevier, Philadelphia.
Figure 6.2: Williams PL, Wendell – Smith CP, Treadgold S (1966) *Basic Human Embryology*, p.78. Lippincott Williams & Wilkins, Baltimore.

8 Microscopic anatomy of the male reproductive tract
Figure 8.1: Bloom W, Fawcett DW (1969) *A Textbook of Histology*, 9th edn, p.688. Saunders/Elsevier.

11 Puberty in boys
Figure 11.1: Marshall WA, Tanner JM (1970) Variations in pattern of pubertal changes in boys. *Arch Dis Child* 45: 13–23.

12 Puberty in girls
Figure 12.1: Marshall WA, Tanner JM (1969) Variations in pattern of pubertal changes in girls. *Arch Dis Child* 44: 291–301.

13 Male reproductive physiology
Figure 13.1(a): Jordan GH (1999) Erectile function and dysfunction. *Postgrad Med 105*: 133.
Figure 13.1(b): Guiliano FA, Rampin O, Benoit G, Jardin A (1995) Neural control of penile erection. *Urol Clin North Am* 22: 748.

16 Fertilization and the establishment of pregnancy
Figure 16.1: Alberts B, Bray D, Lewis J et al. (1994) *Molecular Biology of the Cell*, p.1031. Garland Science/Taylor and Francis, New York.

18 The protein hormones of pregnancy
Figure 18.1(a): Yen SSC (1989) Endocrinology of pregnancy. In: *Maternal–Fetal Medicine* (eds RK Creasy, R Resnik), 2nd edn, p.385. Elsevier, Philadelphia.
Figure 18.1(b): Jaffe RB, (1999) Neuroendocrine-metabolic regulation of pregnancy. In: *Reproductive Endocrinology* (eds SSC Yen, RB Jaffe, RL Barbieri), p.767. Elsevier, Philadelphia.
Figure 18.2: Liu JH, Rebar RW (1999) Endocrinology of pregnancy. In: *Maternal–Fetal Medicine* (eds RK Creasy, R Resnik), 2nd edn, p.386. Elsevier, Philadelphia.

19 The steroid hormones of pregnancy
Figure 19.1: Friesen HG, Cowden EA (1989) Lactation and galactorrhea. In: *Endocrinology* (ed. LJ deGroot), 2nd edn, p.2076. Elsevier.
Figure 19.2: Yen SSC (1989) Endocrinology of pregnancy. In: *Maternal–Fetal Medicine* (eds RK Creasy, R Resnik), 2nd edn, p.377, 380, 382. Elsevier.

26 Abnormalities of male sexual differentiation and development
Figure 26.1: Williams PL, Wendell – Smith CP, Treadgold S (1996) *Basic Human Embryology*, p.81. Lippincott Williams & Wilkins, Baltimore.
Table 26.1: Griffin JE. (1992) Androgen resistance – the clinical and molecular spectrum. *N Eng J Med* 326: 612.

27 Abnormalitites of female sexual differentialtion and development
Figure 27.1: Williams, PL, Wendell – Smith CP, Treadgold S (1966) *Basic Human Embryology*, p.81. Lippincott Williams & Wilkins, Baltimore.

32 Hyperprolactinemia

Figure 32.1: Yen SCC, Jaffe RB (1999) Prolactin in human reproduction. In: *Reproductive Endocrinology* (eds SCC Yen, RB Jaffe, RL Barbieri), p.261. Elsevier.

35 Multifetal pregnancy

Figure 35.1: FitzGerald MJT, FitzGerald M (1994) *Human Embryology*, p.51. Ballière Tindall/Elsevier.

39 Benign and malignant diseases of the breast

Table 39.1: Marchant DJ (1997) *Risk factors in breast disease* (ed. DJ Marchant), pp.116, 119. Elsevier.

41 Diseases of the prostate

Figure 41.1(a): Kirby R, Christmas T (1993) *Anatomy, Embryology and Histopathology in Benign Prostatic Hypertrophy*, p.18. Elsevier.
Figure 41.1(b): Lepor H, Lawson RK, (1993) *Prostate Diseases*, p.45. Elsevier.

42 Ovarian neoplasms

Table 42.1: DiSaia PJ, Creasman RK (1997) Epithelial ovarian cancer. In: *Clinical Gynecologic Oncology*, 5th edn, p.283. Elsevier.

44 Cervical cancer

Figure 44.2: Coleman DV, Evans DMD (1998) *Biopsy Pathology and Cytology of the Cervix*. CRC Press/Taylor and Francis.

46 Sexually transmitted diseases of bacterial origin

Figure 46.1: Diallabetta G, Hook EW, III (1987) Gonococcal infections. *Infect Dis Clin N Amer* 1: 1,28.
Figure 46.2: Batteiger BE, Jones RB (1987) Chlamydial infections. *Infect Dis Clin N Amer* 1: 1,58.

About the companion website

Don't forget to visit the companion website for this book:

www.ataglanceseries.com/reproduction

There you will find valuable material designed to enhance your learning, including:
• Flashcards
• Interactive MCQs from book
• Interactive SAQs

Scan this QR code to visit the companion website:

1 The pituitary gland and gonadotropins

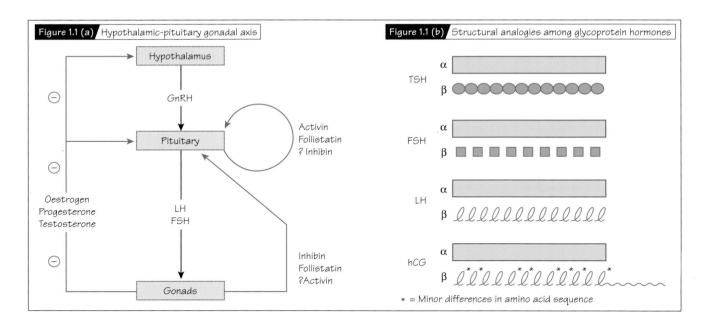

Figure 1.1 (a) Hypothalamic-pituitary gonadal axis

Figure 1.1 (b) Structural analogies among glycoprotein hormones

* = Minor differences in amino acid sequence

Pituitary structure and function

There are three lobes to the pituitary gland (hypophysis): the **anterior lobe**, the **posterior lobe** and the **pars intermedia**, a small intermediate structure lying between the anterior and posterior lobe that is actually a subdivision of the anterior lobe.

The pituitary is connected to the brain via a small branch of tissue known as the pituitary stalk or infundibulum. The posterior pituitary serves mainly as a storage site for two hormones produced in the hypothalamus: oxytocin and arginine vasopressin (also known as antidiuretic hormone, ADH). In contrast, the anterior pituitary produces tropic hormones under the regulatory control of the hypothalamus. This control is mediated by neuroendocrine signals from the hypothalamus that travel through rich vascular connections surrounding the pituitary stalk. Blood flowing through this highly vascular plexus delivers signals to the anterior pituitary gland, regulating production and release of its protein products.

There are five cell types in the anterior pituitary that are associated with tropic hormone production: gonadotropes, lactotropes, somatotropes, thyrotropes and corticotropes. These specific cells are responsible for production and secretion of: **follicle-stimulating hormone (FSH)** and **luteinizing hormone (LH)**; **prolactin**; **growth hormone**; **thyroid-stimulating hormone (TSH)**; and **adrenocorticotropic hormone (ACTH)**, respectively. The thyrotropes and gonadotropes closely resemble each other histologically because their secretory products, LH, FSH and TSH, are all glycoprotein hormones that stain with carbohydrate-sensitive reagents. LH and FSH are produced by a single cell type, allowing coupled secretion and regulation by a single releasing factor.

Control of pituitary gland activity comes largely from the hypothalamus with important direct modulation by feedback mechanisms. The hypothalamic nuclei associated with reproduction include the supraoptic, paraventricular, arcuate, ventromedial and suprachiasmatic nuclei. Neurons in two less well-defined areas, the medial anterior hypothalamus and the medial preoptic areas, are also involved. The magnocellular (large) neurons that originate in the supraoptic and paraventricular nuclei project into the posterior pituitary and produce the hormones vasopressin and oxytocin. The parvocellular (small) neurons found in the paraventricular, arcuate and ventromedial nuclei and the periventricular and medial preoptic areas produce regulatory peptides that control the tropic hormones produced by the anterior pituitary.

Those cells in the hypothalamic nuclei that regulate the pituitary have several functions. They receive signals from higher centers in the brain, generate neural signals of their own and have neuroendocrine capabilities. The higher areas of the brain that connect to the hypothalamic nuclei involved with reproduction are the locus ceruleus, the medulla and pons, the midbrain raphe, the olfactory bulb, the limbic system (amygdala and hippocampus), the piriform cortex and the retina. Endogenous opioids also influence hypothalamic function.

The **neuroendocrine signals** generated within the hypothalamus are mediated by peptide-releasing factors that travel through the hypothalamic–pituitary portal system to their site of action in the pituitary gland. Gonadotropin-releasing hormone (**GnRH**) is the key tropic hormone for regulating gonadotrope cell function and hence, reproduction. A key **neural signal** in human reproduction arises from what is known as the **GnRH pulse generator**. The mechanism by which pulsatile GnRH release controls gonadotropin synthesis and secretion remains poorly defined. At baseline, GnRH secretes from the hypothalamus in pulses at a frequency of approximately one pulse per hour. GnRH pulse frequency is most rapid in the follicular phase, slightly slower in the early luteal phase and slowest in the late luteal phase of the female menstrual cycle. In general, rapid pulse frequencies favor LH secretion and slower pulse frequencies favor FSH release. The

The Reproductive System at a Glance, Fourth Edition. Linda J. Heffner and Danny J. Schust.

relationship between pulse frequency and LH and FSH secretion appears to exist in both women and men. Continuous GnRH release inhibits gonadotrope function. This is the basis for the downregulating activities of long-acting exogenous GnRH agonists and antagonists.

Thyrotropin-releasing hormone (TRH) and **prolactin inhibitory factor (PIF)** also have roles in reproductive regulation. Those hypothalamic neuroendocrine peptides that control growth hormone (GH) and ACTH secretion are less directly related to reproduction.

Structure of LH and FSH

LH, FSH and TSH are structurally similar. They are formed by two distinct, noncovalently bound protein subunits called α and β. The pregnancy-specific gonadotropin, human chorionic gonadotropin (hCG), is a fourth glycoprotein formed of α and β chains. The α subunit for all four hormones is identical. The β subunit of each hormone differs, conferring functional specificity on each $\alpha\beta$ dimer (Fig. 1.1a and b). The β chains for LH and hCG are the most similar with 82% homology. Carbohydrate side chains on both the α and β chains of LH, hCG and FSH add to structural specificity. The carbohydrate chains also influence metabolic clearance rates for the glycoprotein hormones. This effect is most dramatic with the hCG molecule. The β chain of hCG has a 24 amino acid extension at its C terminus that contains four O-linked polysaccharides. This sugar-laden "tail" dramatically slows the clearance of hCG. By prolonging its half-life, the effects of small amounts of this glycoprotein are dramatically enhanced. This characteristic is very important in early pregnancy recognition and maintenance (Chapters 16 and 18).

Regulation of FSH and LH

The biosynthesis and secretion of FSH and LH are tightly controlled within the reproductive cycle. There are multiple ways in which FSH and LH can be regulated, including alterations in gene transcription, mRNA stabilization, rate of protein subunit synthesis, posttranslational glycosylation and changes in the number of gonadotropin-secreting cells.

Gonadal steroids exert negative feedback control over FSH and LH synthesis and secretion. Estrogen, androgen and progesterone receptors are present in the gonadotropin-secreting cells of the pituitary and in some neurons in the hypothalamus. In the pituitary, the gonadal steroids appear to affect the transcription rate of the genes coding for FSH-β, LH-β and the common α subunit. While there is some evidence that steroids can act at the level of the hypothalamic pulse generator, gonadal steroid hormone receptors do not appear to be present in the GnRH-containing cells of the arcuate nucleus.

There is one important exception to the generally inhibitory effect of gonadal steroids on gonadotrope function. In certain situations, estrogen exerts positive feedback on gonadotropin secretion. This is critical to produce the midcycle LH surge in women (Chapter 14) and requires a sustained (>48 h) elevation in circulating estradiol. Estrogen-induced stimulation involves both increased gonadotropin gene expression in the pituitary and alterations in GnRH pulse frequency in the hypothalamus.

Inhibin and **activin** are closely related peptides produced by the ovary, testes, pituitary gland and placenta that influence gonadotrope function. As suggested by their names, inhibin decreases gonadotrope function and activin stimulates it. Inhibin and activin are formed from common α and β subunits. Inhibin is formed of one α subunit linked to either of two highly homologous β subunits to form inhibin A ($\alpha\beta_A$) or inhibin B ($\alpha\beta_B$). Activin is composed of three combinations of the β subunits: activin A ($\beta_A\beta_A$), activin AB ($\beta_A\beta_B$) and activin B ($\beta_B\beta_B$). Activin is a member of the transforming growth factor β (TGF-β) superfamily of growth and differentiation factors that include TGF-β, Müllerian-inhibiting substance (MIS) and bone morphogenic proteins. **Follistatin** is structurally unrelated to either inhibin or activin. It is a highly glycosylated pituitary peptide that inhibits gonadotrope function at one-third the potency of inhibin. All three of these peptides have their major influence on the expression of the FSH-β gene. Of these peptides, inhibin appears to be the most biologically important regulator of the FSH gene, directly suppressing its activity. The other two peptides appear to act within the pituitary cells through locally released second messengers or autocrine peptides. Activin B stimulates FSH release. Activins also affect the gonads directly by increasing the activity of the aromatase enzyme in the ovary and stimulating proliferation of spermatogonia in the testes.

Mechanism of action of gonadotropins

There are distinct FSH and LH **receptors**. The latter also bind the closely related hCG molecule. Receptors for both glycoprotein hormones FSH and LH are located in the plasma membranes of the granulosa cells in the ovary and the Sertoli cells in the testes. Ovarian thecal cells and testicular Leydig cells only display LH receptors. In addition to regulating steroidogenesis and gametogenesis, gonadotropins regulate expression of their own receptors in a dose-dependent fashion. FSH also induces LH/hCG receptor formation in granulosa and Sertoli cells.

Although gonadotropin receptors are normally present in very low concentrations on the cell surface, they have high specificity and affinity for their ligands. The interactions between the glycoprotein dimer and its receptor lead to conformational changes in the receptor. This then activates a membrane-associated **G protein-coupled signaling system**. Although the G protein-coupled cAMP pathway is the principal mediator of both FSH and LH receptor activity, activation of the protein kinase C system can also occur.

In addition to activating specific intracellular signaling processes, binding of the gonadotropin to its receptor also initiates a regulatory function termed **desensitization**. Desensitization reduces the cell's responsiveness to ongoing stimulation. In the first phase of desensitization, the gonadotropin receptor becomes "uncoupled" from its downstream activity so that it no longer activates adenylate cyclase. In the second, slower phase of desensitization, the degradation rate for the receptors is increased. This latter process is called "downregulation." Both are involved in the activities of GnRH agonists and antagonists.

2 Steroid hormone biosynthesis

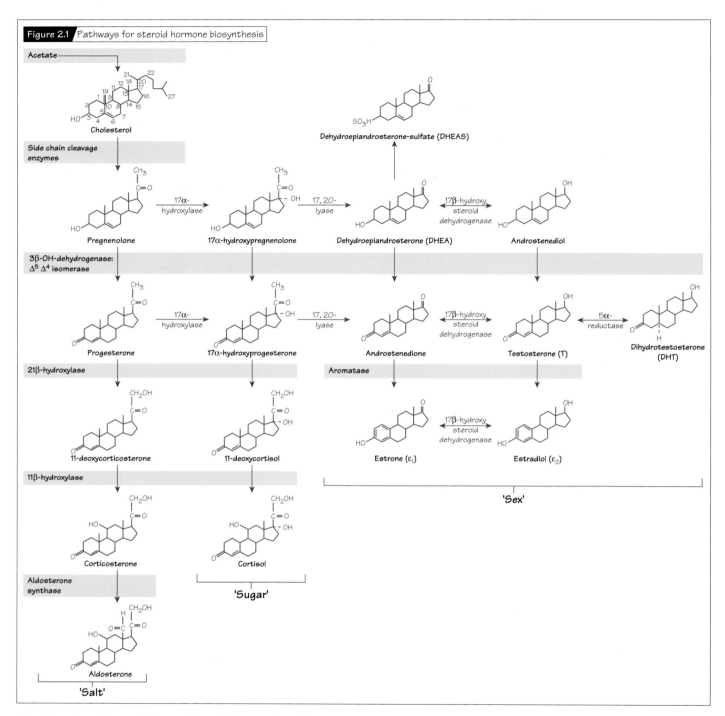

Figure 2.1 Pathways for steroid hormone biosynthesis

Cholesterol and the steroid production pathway

Cholesterol is the building block of steroid hormones. All steroid-producing organs with the exception of the placenta can synthesize cholesterol from acetate. Under most circumstances, however, local synthesis cannot meet demand and circulating cholesterol must be used. The major carriers of cholesterol in the bloodstream are the **low-density lipoproteins (LDLs)**. LDL is removed from the blood by steroidogenic cells using cell surface receptors that recognize specific surface proteins on LDL called apoproteins. Once in the cell, cholesterol is carried through a sequence of enzymatic changes to produce a final product that belongs to one of the major classes of steroid hormones: progestins, androgens and estrogens (sex), glucocorticoids (sugar) and mineralocorticoids (salt). All steroid-producing tissues use

The Reproductive System at a Glance, Fourth Edition. Linda J. Heffner and Danny J. Schust.

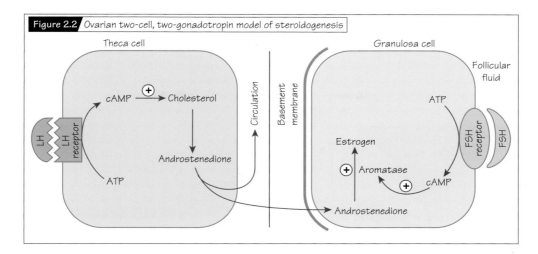

Figure 2.2 Ovarian two-cell, two-gonadotropin model of steroidogenesis

a common sequence of precursor molecules and enzymes (Fig. 2.1). Tissue specificity is conferred by the presence or absence of specific enzymes in the sequence. For instance, the gonads differ from the adrenal glands in that ovaries and testes do not express the 21-hydroxylase or 11β-hydroxylase enzymes that are necessary to produce corticosteroids. Therefore, the gonads only produce three classes of steroids: progestins, androgens and estrogens.

During conversion of cholesterol to steroid metabolites, the number of total carbon atoms decreases sequentially. Progestins have 21 carbons (C-21); androgens have 19 carbons (C-19); and estrogens have 18 carbons (C-18). Thus, progestins are obligatory precursors of both androgens and estrogens. Likewise, androgens are obligatory precursors of estrogens.

Most of the steroidogenic enzymes are members of the **cytochrome P450 class of oxidases**. A single mitochondrial protein P450scc, the cholesterol side chain cleavage enzyme, mediates all steps in the conversion of cholesterol to pregnenolone. The activity of this protein represents the rate-limiting step for the entire steroid pathway. Not surprisingly, it is also the major site of tropic hormone stimulation. Genetic mutations of P450scc are very rare and usually lethal. No steroid hormones can be produced by an individual with an inactive P450scc enzyme.

Once pregnenolone is formed, steroid production can proceed down one of two paths, through either progesterone or 17α-hydroxypregnenolone. All but two of the enzymes responsible for producing the steroid hormones are packaged within the endoplasmic reticulum, together with other members of the P450 system. The biosynthetic units are very tightly linked together, thereby ensuring that very few of the steroid intermediates leave the cell. This packaging is also highly efficient in that it can convert an entire class of steroids to another. Thus, 17,20-desmolase will convert all progestins to androgens, and aromatase will convert all androgens but dihydrotestosterone (DHT) to estrogens.

Sites of production

Ovary

In the ovary, steroid production occurs in a **two-cell system** (Fig. 2.2). Theca cells produce androgens. These androgens diffuse into the granulosa cells where they are converted to estrogens. Tropic hormones regulate specific steps in the sex steroid cascade. Theca cells respond to **luteinizing hormone (LH)** by increasing the number of LDL receptors and hence cholesterol entry into the cells. LH also stimulates P450scc

activity, allowing increased androgen production. When these androgens diffuse into granulosa cells, they are metabolized by aromatase into estrogens. **Follicle-stimulating hormone (FSH)** induces the activity of aromatase in the granulosa cell, thereby increasing the conversion of androgens to estrogens. The single aromatase gene has many promoter sites. These are responsive to cytokines, cyclic nucleotides, gonadotropins, glucocorticoids and growth factors.

Testes

In the testes, androgen production occurs largely in the Leydig cells under the influence of LH. Androgens produced in the Leydig cells either enter the bloodstream directly or diffuse into nearby Sertoli cells. Sertoli cells can convert androgens to estrogens using aromatase or reduce them to dihydrotestosterone via 5α-reductase. Because the specific cell types within the differentiated male and female gonads have common embryonic origins (Chapter 5), the mechanisms for steroid production in the testes very much parallel those in the ovary.

Adrenals

Sex hormone production by the adrenals occurs largely as a by-product of corticosteroid biosynthesis. The contribution of adrenal sex steroids to the total pool of circulating sex steroids is typically small, although there are several important exceptions. The ovaries of postmenopausal women no longer produce significant amounts of steroid hormones so adrenal androgen production can become clinically significant. In pregnancy, the placenta cannot synthesize cholesterol from acetate. Rather, it relies on adrenal androgens of both maternal and fetal origin to make estrogens.

With the exception of P450scc, inherited defects in any of the enzymes involved in steroidogenesis are associated with clinical syndromes resulting either from accumulation of a precursor product or absence of a key end-product. For example, an inherited deficiency of the enzyme 21-hydroxylase in the adrenal gland will lead to a deficiency in adrenal cortisol production. Low cortisol levels feed back to promote enhanced production of adrenal glucocorticoids. The enzymatic block, however, results in an accumulation of precursor progestins, some of which will be shunted down functional androgen biosynthetic pathways. If the 21-hydroxylase deficiency occurs in a female fetus, the increase in androgen production may cause masculinization of the external genitalia, known as congenital adrenal hyperplasia syndrome (Chapter 27). Similarly, disorders of male sexual differentiation and development may result from genetic defects in androgen production (Chapter 26).

3 Steroid hormone mechanism of action and metabolism

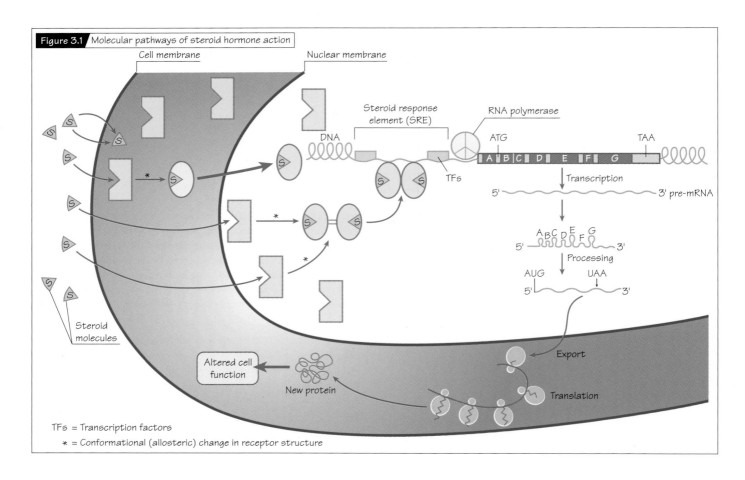

Figure 3.1 Molecular pathways of steroid hormone action

TFs = Transcription factors

* = Conformational (allosteric) change in receptor structure

Mechanisms of steroid action

Steroid hormones exert their effects via a unifying basic mechanism: the induction of new protein synthesis in their target cells. These induced proteins may be hormones themselves or other molecules important to cell function, such as enzymes. It is the newly synthesized proteins that are ultimately responsible for steroid hormone activity (Fig. 3.1).

Once a steroid hormone is secreted by its endocrine gland of origin, 95–98% of it circulates in the bloodstream bound to a specific transport protein. The remaining 2–5% is free to diffuse into all cells. Once inside the cell, a steroid can only produce responses in cells that have **specific intracellular receptors** for that hormone. Specific receptor binding is key to the action of steroids in their target tissues. Thus, estrogen receptors are found in the brain and in target cells specific to female reproduction, such as the uterus and breast. Facial hair follicles and penile erectile tissue contain androgen receptors. Glucocorticoid receptors are found in all cells because glucocorticoids are necessary to regulate global functions like metabolism and stress.

All members of the major classes of sex steroids (e.g., androgens, estrogens and progestins) act through a similar sequence of events to exert cellular responses: (i) transfer of the steroid into the nucleus; (ii) intranuclear receptor binding; (iii) alterations in receptor conformation that convert the receptor from an inactive to an active form; (iv) binding of the steroid–receptor complex to regulatory elements on deoxyribonucleic acid (DNA); (v) transcription and synthesis of new messenger ribonucleic acid (mRNA); and (vi) translation of mRNA with new protein synthesis in the cell. The mechanisms of action of glucocorticoids and mineralocorticoids differ from those of the sex steroids. Glucocorticoids and mineralocorticoids bind to their receptors in the cell cytoplasm. Hormone–receptor complexes are subsequently transported to the nucleus where they bind to the DNA.

There are three important structural domains in each steroid hormone receptor that correspond to the molecule's three functions: (i) steroid hormone binding; (ii) DNA binding; and (iii) promotion of gene transcription. It is therefore not surprising that all steroid hormone receptors have remarkable structural similarities at the copy DNA (cDNA) level. The receptors for thyroid hormone, vitamin D and vitamin A also have similar DNA binding domains. Together with the sex hormone receptors, these receptors form a "superfamily" of nuclear receptors in which the thyroid hormone and vitamin A and D receptors are thought to be the most evolutionarily primitive. The latter three receptors are highly conserved, likely a result of their importance in early embryonic development. Glucocorticoid and progesterone receptors arose more recently in evolution. Their actions are less global, regulating acute metabolic changes in highly differentiated cells.

The Reproductive System at a Glance, Fourth Edition. Linda J. Heffner and Danny J. Schust.

Expression of genes regulated by steroid hormones is controlled by four specific elements: (i) promoters; (ii) steroid-responsive enhancers; (iii) silencers; and (iv) hormone-independent enhancers. Steroid-responsive enhancers are DNA binding sites for activated steroid–receptor complexes and are known as steroid response elements (SREs). SREs are a very important component of hormone-responsive genes; they determine steroid specificity.

Agonists and antagonists

Steroid hormone potency depends on a combination of the affinity of the receptor for the hormone or drug, the affinity of the hormone–receptor complex for the SRE, and the efficiency of the activated hormone–receptor complex in regulating gene transcription. Molecules with high affinities for a receptor and whose subsequent hormone–receptor complex has high affinity for an SRE lead to prolonged occupancy of the SRE and sustained gene transcription. Such molecules act as agonists for the parent compound. Other molecules may have a high affinity for a receptor, but the hormone–receptor complex binds inefficiently to the SRE. Still others occupy the steroid receptor in a way that allows them to bind to the SRE but prevents RNA polymerase from coupling with factors necessary for gene transcription. The latter act as antagonists to the parent compound. An example of a compound with mixed agonist/antagonist properties is the drug tamoxifen. **Tamoxifen** is an antiestrogen that acts as a potent antagonist to the estrogen receptor in breast tissue and as an agonist in uterus and bone. Such tissue-specific effects are dependent upon specific silencers and hormone-independent enhancers present in each tissue. Another widely used agonist/antagonist is the non-steroidal compound clomiphene citrate. **Clomiphene** can be used to induce ovulation, although its actions are complex. Clomiphene's interactions with estrogen receptors in the pituitary gland and hypothalamus result in binding of receptors, but without subsequent efficient stimulation of estrogen-associated gene transcription. The hypothalamus senses this as a hypo-estrogenic state and gonadotropin-releasing hormone (GnRH) pulse frequency increases. Pituitary follicle-stimulating hormone (FSH) production is stimulated and increased FSH release drives ovarian production of estrogen. When clomiphene is stopped, the hypothalamic estrogen receptors are again available for estrogen binding and appropriate SRE responses. The hypothalamus is able to respond normally to the high concentrations of circulating estrogen from the ovaries and an ovulatory luteinizing hormone (LH) surge occurs (Chapter 14).

Steroids in the circulation

Steroid hormones are transported in the bloodstream bound to specific proteins. Protein-bound hormone does not traverse the plasma membrane of the cell. Nearly 70% of circulating testosterone and estradiol is bound to a β globulin known as **sex hormone-binding globulin (SHBG)**. Another 30% is loosely bound to albumin, leaving only 1–2% unbound and capable of entering cells. SHBG binds all other estrogens and androgens to varying degrees; less than 10% of any steroid is free in the bloodstream. Pregnancy, estrogen and hyperthyroidism all increase SHBG synthesis. Androgens, progestins, corticoids and growth hormone all decrease SHBG. Weight gain can also decrease SHBG through an insulin-mediated effect on its synthesis. In keeping with the law of mass action, changes in the concentration of SHBG will affect the amount of free, unbound circulating steroid. Changes in SHBG will therefore affect the biologic action of steroids by altering the amount available to cells.

Unlike the other sex steroids, progesterone is carried in the blood by a glycoprotein, corticosteroid-binding globulin (CBG). CBG is also known as transcortin. As suggested by its name, it binds and carries glucocorticoids.

Steroid metabolism

With the exception of the progestins, androgens are obligatory precursors of all other steroid hormones. Therefore, androgens are made in all steroid-producing tissues including the testis, ovary and adrenal gland. The major circulating androgen in men is testosterone which is produced by the testes. **Testosterone is the most potent androgen**. Its hormonal action is produced either directly through binding to the androgen receptor or indirectly after **conversion to dihydrotestosterone (DHT)** within the target tissue. Testosterone acts directly on the internal genital tract in male fetuses during sexual differentiation (Chapter 6) and on skeletal muscle to promote growth. DHT acts on the genital tracts of male fetuses to stimulate differentiation of the external genitalia. In adult men, DHT acts locally to maintain masculinized external genitalia and secondary sexual characteristics such as facial and pubic hair. Other major circulating androgens in men include androstenedione, androstenediol, dehydroepiandrosterone (DHEA) and dehydroepiandrosterone sulfate (DHEA-S).

All of the above androgens, including testosterone and DHT, can be found in the circulation of women. With the exception of androstenedione, the concentrations of the androgens are considerably lower in women than in men. Androstenedione is unique in that only about 4% of it is bound to SHBG in the circulation in women. The remainder is bound more loosely to albumin. Circulating androstenedione functions largely as a prohormone and is converted within target tissues to testosterone, estrone and estradiol.

Estradiol (E_2) is the major estrogen secreted by the ovary. Estrone (E_1) is also secreted by the ovary in significant amounts. Estriol (E_3), by contrast, is not produced in the ovary at all. Estriol is produced from estradiol and estrone in peripheral tissues and from androgen in the placenta; it is considered a less active "metabolite" of the more potent estrogens. Direct conversion of androgens into estrone can occur in skin and adipose tissue. This has important clinical implications in the obese female. In all women, the daily production of the prohormone androstenedione is 10 times higher than that of estradiol. In obese women, conversion of androgens to estrone in adipose tissue can become a major source of excessive amounts of circulating estrogen.

The adrenal gland is an important source of sex steroids in both men and women. Androstenedione, DHEA and DHEA-S are the major circulating androgens of adrenal origin and adrenal androgen production follows a circadian rhythm that parallels cortisol secretion. Adrenal androgens assume an important role in the postmenopausal woman. In the absence of ovarian estrogen production, adrenal androgens act as a major source for estrogen precursors.

The most abundant progestin in the circulation is **progesterone**. The ovary, testis, placenta and adrenal gland can all produce progesterone. 17-Hydroxyprogesterone of adrenal and ovarian origin represents the other major circulating progestin. Both progestins are largely bound by transcortin.

Steroid excretion

Steroids are excreted in urine and bile. Prior to elimination, most active steroids are conjugated as either sulfates or glucuronides. Some sulfated conjugates such as DHEA-S are actively secreted. These conjugated hormones can serve as precursors to active hormone metabolites in target tissues that have the enzymes to hydrolyze the ester bonds involved in the conjugation.

4 Reproductive genetics

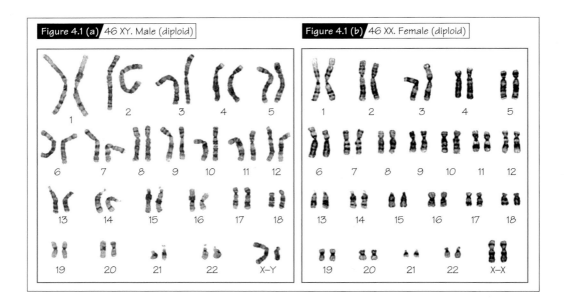

Figure 4.1 (a) 46 XY. Male (diploid)

Figure 4.1 (b) 46 XX. Female (diploid)

Chromosomes

Human chromosomes are complex structures consisting of deoxyribo-nucleic acid (DNA), ribonucleic acid (RNA) and protein. Each single helix of DNA is bound at each end with a telomere and has a centro-mere somewhere along the length of the chromosome. The telomere protects the ends of the chromosome during DNA replication. Tel-omere shortening is associated with aging. The centromere is the site at which the mitotic spindle will attach and is necessary for proper segregation of chromosomes during cell division. The centromere divides the chromosome into two arms, identified as p (petit) for the short arm and q for the long arm. The centromere can be positioned anywhere along the arm of the chromosome and its location has been used to group like chromosomes together as central (metacentric), distal (acrocentric) or others (submetacentric). The length of the chro-mosome plus the position of its centromere are used to identify indi-vidual chromosomes within the 22 pairs of autosomes and one pair of sex chromosomes. Chromosomes are numbered in descending order of size; 1 is the largest. The only exception to this rule is chromosomes 21 and 22; 22 is larger than 21. Because of the historical convention of associating Down syndrome with trisomy 21, this chromosome pair was not renamed when the size difference became apparent.

A **karyotype** is a display of chromosomes ordered from 1 to 22 plus the sex chromosomes, with each chromosome oriented so that the p arm is on top. Females have a 46XX karyotype and males a 46XY karyotype (Fig. 4.1a and b).

Mitosis and meiosis

These are two distinct types of cell divisions, with several common features. The first is the need to duplicate the entire chromosome content of the cell prior to division. Both also use the cell machinery of the parent cell to make the DNA, RNA and new proteins that will participate in the cell division. Finally, both processes rely on using the mitotic spindle to separate the chromosomes into the two poles of the cell that are destined to become the progeny of that cell. Mitosis

and meiosis differ in that duplicated chromosomes behave differently after DNA replication (Fig. 4.2). In mitosis, there is no difference in total chromosome content between parent and daughter cells; in meiosis, the chromosome number of the daughter cells is eventually reduced from 46 to 23, which is necessary to convert the diploid germ cell precursors originating in the embryo into haploid ($1n$) germ cells. These haploid germ cells will produce a new diploid organism at fertilization. Meiosis promotes exchange of genetic material through chromatid crossing over; mitosis does not.

During the **interphase** preceding cell division, the DNA for each chromosome is duplicated to $4n$. Thus, each chromosome consists of two identical **chromatids** joined at the centromere.

In mitosis, the chromosomes first shorten and thicken and the nucle-oli and nuclear membrane break down (**prophase**). During **met-aphase**, a mitotic spindle forms between the two centrioles of the cell and all chromosomes line up on its equator. The centromere of each chromosome splits and one chromatid from each chromosome migrates to the polar ends of the mitotic spindle (**anaphase**). In **telophase**, new nucleoli and nuclear membranes form, the parent cell divides into two daughter cells and the mitotic spindle is disassembled. Two genetically identical cells now exist in place of the parent cell. **Mitosis is a non-sexual or vegetative form of reproduction**.

Meiosis involves two sequential cell divisions, again beginning with the $4n$ DNA produced in interphase. In prophase of the first division (**prophase 1**), several specific and recognizable events occur. In the **leptotene** stage, the chromosomes become barely visible as long thin structures. Homologous pairs of chromosomes then come to lie side by side along parts of their length, forming tetrads (**zygotene** stage). The chromosomes thicken and shorten, much as they do in mitotic prophase (**pachytene** stage); however, the pairing that occurred in the zygotene stage allows **synapsis**, **crossing-over** and **chromatid exchange** to happen. In the **diplotene/diakinesis** stage, the chromo-somes shorten even more. The paired homologous chromosomes show evidence of the crossing-over and chromatid exchange, displaying

The Reproductive System at a Glance, Fourth Edition. Linda J. Heffner and Danny J. Schust.

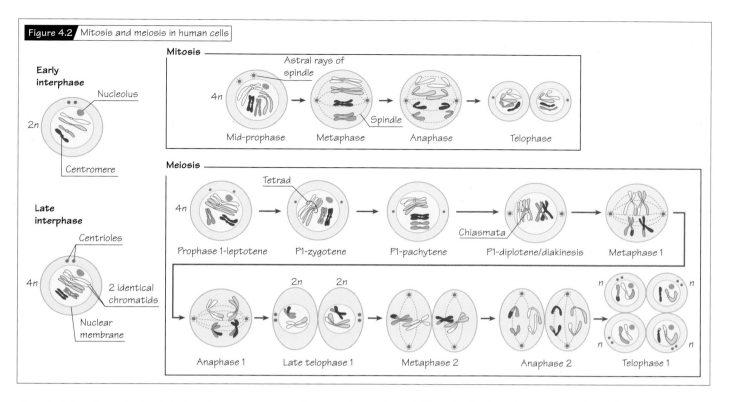

Figure 4.2 Mitosis and meiosis in human cells

characteristic chiasmata that join the chromosome arms. Loops and unusual shapes within the chromosomes may be apparent at this stage. In **metaphase 1** of meiosis, the nuclear membrane breaks down and the joined pairs of homologous chromosomes line up at the equator of the spindle apparatus. One of each pair of homologous chromosomes then moves to each end of the cell along the spindle (**anaphase 1**). Nuclear membranes may then form, yielding two haploid daughter cells with 23 $2n$ chromosomes in **telophase 1**. In the second meiotic division, these haploid cells divide as if in mitosis. This second division produces four haploid cells each containing 23 $1n$ chromosomes. **Unlike the cells produced in mitosis, these daughter germ cells are genetically unique and different from the parent cells because of the genetic exchanges that took place in the diplotene stage.** Haploid germ cells participate in sexual reproduction in which a sperm cell and oocyte come together to form a new diploid zygote.

While the sequence of events in meiosis during spermatogenesis and oogenesis is basically the same, there are several important differences. In the prepubertal male, primordial germ cells are arrested in interphase. At puberty, these cells are reactivated to enter rounds of mitoses in the basal compartment of the seminiferous tubule. These reactivated cells are known as spermatogonial stem cells. From this reservoir of stem cells, early spermatogonia emerge and divide several times again to produce a "clone" of spermatogonia with identical genotypes. All the spermatogonia from the clone then enter meiosis 1 and 2 to produce unique haploid sperm. New stem cells are constantly entering the spermatogenic cycle (Chapter 8) and thus the sperm supply is constantly renewing itself. Because of the relatively short time for spermatocytes to progress through meiosis and because of the tremendous competition among spermatozoa to reach the single oocyte within the female tract, fertilization of an egg by an aneuploid sperm is far rarer than the converse.

In contrast to the testis, the ovary of a female at birth contains all the germ cells it will ever have. These oocytes remain arrested in prophase 1 of meiosis until the LH surge at ovulation initiates met-aphase 1. Thus, the duplicated genetic material within the oocyte exists paired with its homologous chromosome for 10–50 years before the cell is called upon to divide. For this reason alone, oocytes are much more prone to chromosome abnormalities than are sperm.

Non-disjunction

This is the failure of a chromosome pair to separate during meiosis, and can occur at either meiosis 1 or 2. When a single chromosome is involved, the aneuploid zygote is either **monosomic** or **trisomic** for the chromosome pair that failed to divide properly. With the exception of monosomy X or Turner syndrome, monosomic embryos are uniformly miscarried (Chapter 36). Most trisomic fetuses are also miscarried; only three (trisomy 13, 18 and 21) are reported among live births. Those that survive to birth are likely mosaics that carry nonaffected cell lineages. If all the chromosomes are present in multiples other than $2n$, the embryo or fetus is **polyploid**.

Imprinting

Although it is critical that the zygote has $2n$ chromosomes, it is also important that one set of chromosomes comes from each parent. Dermoid cysts and hydatidiform moles (gestational trophoblastic disease; Chapter 45) each have all 46 chromosomes from a single parent. Cytogenetic studies of these entities have shown the importance of imprinting in early embryonic development. Imprinting is the process by which specific genes are methylated so that they can no longer be transcribed. Normal embryonic development requires that one set of genes be maternally imprinted and a second paternally. Otherwise, important steps in development will not occur and the zygote cannot form normally. For instance, two sets of maternally imprinted genes are present in dermoid tumors of the ovary, resulting in development of disorganized fetal tissues without any supporting placenta or fetal membranes. Conversely, two sets of paternally imprinted genes are present in hydatidiform moles. In these cases, dysplastic trophoblast develops, but a fetus does not.

5 Gonadal development in the embryo

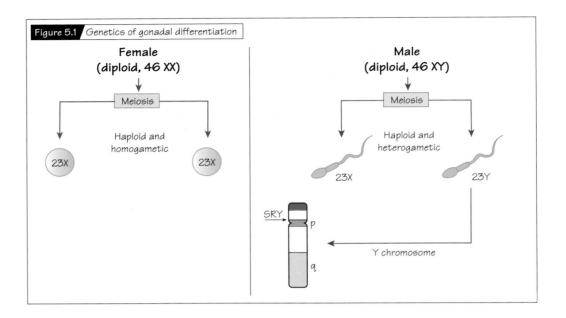

Figure 5.1 Genetics of gonadal differentiation

Female (diploid, 46 XX) → Meiosis → Haploid and homogametic → 23X, 23X

Male (diploid, 46 XY) → Meiosis → Haploid and heterogametic → 23X, 23Y

SRY — p, q — Y chromosome

Role of sex chromatin in reproductive development

All mammalian females are homogametic and represent the "default" pathway in sexual differentiation. Homogametic describes the sex whose cell nuclei contain two similar sex chromosomes. While this characterizes mammalian females, the homogametic sex is male in butterflies, birds and some amphibians and fishes. In humans, all normal oocytes from genetic females will carry 22 autosomes and an X chromosome (22X). Mammalian embryos of both genetic sexes are bathed in relatively large amounts of placental estrogen during development. In the absence of specific factors regulated by a single gene on the Y chromosome, embryos will develop into a female phenotype. The human female, like all mammalian females, represents the fundamental or undifferentiated phenotypic sex.

All mammalian males are heterogametic. They produce gametes with both 22X and 22Y chromosome complements. Males are considered the differentiated phenotypic sex. With few exceptions, any individual that carries a specific piece of the Y chromosome will develop a testis and a male phenotype. This segment of the Y chromosome has been called the **sex-determining region of the Y chromosome (SRY)** (Fig. 5.1). Specific instruction from the SRY region of the Y chromosome directs the undifferentiated gonad to become a testis. **Without the presence of SRY, a fetus will develop along the default or female phenotypic pathway**.

The Y chromosome is much smaller than the X and very little of its DNA is available for RNA synthesis. Many of the genes that control testicular development from the undifferentiated gonad are therefore located on other chromosomes, including autosomes and the X chromosome. However, the Y chromosomecontains a specific, single-copy gene that determines testicular differentiation. This gene is located on the short arm of the chromosome within SRY and appears to activate genes on other chromosomes.

Evidence for the importance of SRY comes from both clinical and experimental research results. Examination of the DNA sequences of women with XY karyotypes has revealed that a single locus within the Y chromosome must be present and intact for an individual to have a testis. Absence of, or damage to, this DNA sequence in individuals with an otherwise intact 46XY male chromosomal content results in ovarian development and a phenotypic female. Likewise, examination of the DNA sequences of phenotypic men with XX karyotypes will reveal the aberrant presence of SRY sequences.

Gonadal differentiation

Gonadal development begins in the human at the 4th embryonic (6th menstrual) week in parallel with the formation of the ventral body wall. The first step in gonadal development is the migration of undifferentiated primordial germ cells from their site of formation in the yolk sac. These germ cells arise from the endoderm lining the yolk sac; they detach themselves and migrate dorsally along the yolk stalk, midgut and dorsal mesentery to reach the genital ridges. The genital ridges lie on the medial aspect of the mesonephric ridge that will contribute to the developing kidney. Over the next 2 weeks the primordial germ cells mitose repeatedly, forming a vast population of precursor gametes. Failure of these germ cells to develop and populate the genital ridges at this time will result in complete failure of gonadal formation.

When germ cells reach the coelomic epithelium lining the genital ridge, cellular contact causes the coelomic epithelia to differentiate into a primitive germinal epithelium. The germ cells become embedded in the primitive germinal epithelium during this process of differentiation. This combination of germinal epithelia and germ cells forms the sex cords. The connection of the sex cords to the coelomic wall (gonadal surface) is maintained at this point. The gonads are now histologically distinct, bipotent organs that may become testes or

The Reproductive System at a Glance, Fourth Edition. Linda J. Heffner and Danny J. Schust.

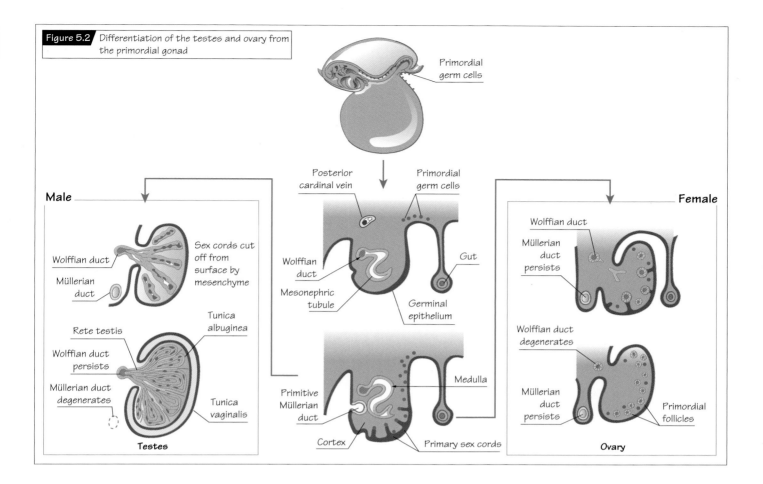

Figure 5.2 Differentiation of the testes and ovary from the primordial gonad

ovaries (Fig. 5.2). Inappropriate or incomplete developmental signals during this stage can result in the rare condition of hermaphroditism. True hermaphrodites have both ovaries and testes and are extremely rare in humans.

In a genetic male, gene products directed by activation of the SRY locus on the Y chromosome now cause the undifferentiated sex cords to enlarge, split and begin to form the **primitive testis**. Subepithelial mesenchyme arises between the germinal epithelium and the sex cords and cuts the cords off from the gonadal surface. The sex cords are now housed within the inner portion of the gonad – **the testicular medulla**. The primordial germ cells within the sex cords begin to differentiate into immature sperm cells called **spermatogonia**. The supporting sex cord cells form precursor **Sertoli cells**.

Ovarian differentiation occurs about 2 weeks later than testicular development. Initially, the sex cords of the developing ovary continue to proliferate while maintaining their connection with the gonadal surface. The germ cells begin to differentiate into primordial **oocytes** called oogonia within follicles. The epithelium surrounding the oogonia differentiates into **granulosa cells**. Subepithelial mesenchyme then invades the gonad and breaks up the sex cords, isolating

the follicles. This mesenchyme will become the ovarian stroma. Unlike the testis, developing ovarian gametes are now housed in the outer portion of the gonad – **the ovarian cortex**.

The ovary and testes can be histologically distinguished from each other by the 8th embryonic (10th menstrual) week of pregnancy. The progeny of the germinal epithelium are now apparent as Sertoli cells in the male and granulosa cells in the female. Similarities between males and females in the endocrine function of these cells stem from their common ancestry. The mesenchyme arising beneath the germinal epithelium in the testis is the anlagen of testicular interstitial cells, also known as **Leydig cells**. The mesenchyme arising beneath the germinal epithelium of the ovary is the anlagen of ovarian stroma or **thecal cells**. Functional similarities in these two cell types will also be seen in the mature glands.

Once the undifferentiated gonads begin to develop into either ovaries or testes, the remainder of sexual differentiation is dependent on secretory products of the testes only. In the absence of these specific testicular secretions, the phenotype that develops is completely female. The ovary and its secretory products do not contribute to the development of the uterus, fallopian tubes, vagina or vulva.

6 Phenotypic sex differentiation

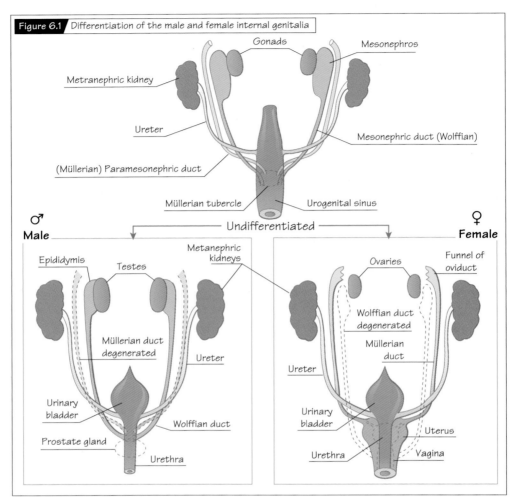

Figure 6.1 Differentiation of the male and female internal genitalia

Undifferentiated:
- Gonads
- Mesonephros
- Metranephric kidney
- Ureter
- Mesonephric duct (Wolffian)
- (Müllerian) Paramesonephric duct
- Müllerian tubercle
- Urogenital sinus

♂ Male:
- Epididymis
- Testes
- Metanephric kidneys
- Müllerian duct degenerated
- Ureter
- Urinary bladder
- Wolffian duct
- Prostate gland
- Urethra

♀ Female:
- Ovaries
- Funnel of oviduct
- Wolffian duct degenerated
- Müllerian duct
- Ureter
- Urinary bladder
- Uterus
- Urethra
- Vagina

Internal genitalia

Unlike the bipotential gonads and external genitalia, the male and female internal genitalia arise from separate duct systems (Fig. 6.1). Development of these structures occurs in parallel and in close physical proximity with the developing urinary system. Both begin to occur at about 4 embryonic (6 menstrual) weeks. The primordial kidney (mesonephros) is composed of tubules and a duct known as the **mesonephric** or **Wolffian duct**. The Wolffian duct grows out from the tubules toward the urogenital sinus. The mesonephric tubules make contact with the primitive sex cords just as the gonad begins to differentiate. Simultaneously, an inpocketing of the coelomic epithelium near the lateral edge of the mesonephric ridge forms the paramesonephric or **Müllerian duct**. As kidney development proceeds (metanephric stage), the mesonephric structures will become totally incorporated into the reproductive tract and lose their urinary function. The Wolffian and Müllerian ducts are primordia for the internal organs of reproduction in the male and female, respectively. In each sex, the other duct system typically disappears by the 3rd fetal month, leaving behind vestiges that are usually unimportant clinically.

In the normal male embryo, the secretion of a peptide called Müllerian-inhibiting substance (MIS; also known as anti-Mullerian hormone or AMH) occurs under the direction of sex-determining region of the Y chromosome (SRY). MIS is secreted by cells that will become Sertoli cells in the adult testis. MIS causes the Müllerian duct to degenerate. Testosterone is produced by those testicular cells destined to become Leydig cells in the adult. Testosterone directs development of the **Wolffian duct system** to form the **epididymis, vas deferens** and **seminal vesicles**. In contrast to the adult, testosterone production by the embryonic testes is controlled not by the hypothalamic–pituitary system, but by the placental hormone human chorionic gonadotropin (hCG).

The absence of MIS in the female embryo permits the Müllerian system to persist. Upon reaching the urogenital sinus, the Müllerian ducts induce the formation of a vaginal plate. Contact of the Müllerian ducts with the vaginal plate also initiates the fusion of the ducts to form the body of the uterus. The Müllerian ducts will form the **fallopian tubes, uterus** and the **upper portion of the vagina**. Failure of the Müllerian ducts to develop or fuse completely can cause uterine and cervical anomalies. In the absence of testosterone, the Wolffian system regresses. A vestige of the Wolffian duct, known as Gartner's duct, persists in its length from the ovary to the hymen. Clinically apparent cysts may form anywhere along Gartner's duct.

The Reproductive System at a Glance, Fourth Edition. Linda J. Heffner and Danny J. Schust.

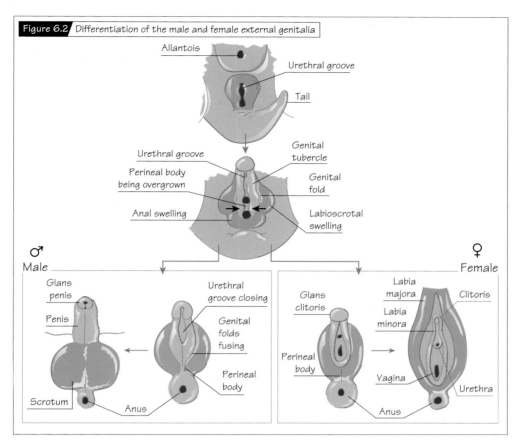

Figure 6.2 Differentiation of the male and female external genitalia

Most of the **prostate gland** develops from the same primordial area of the urogenital sinus that forms the vaginal plate in the female, making the prostate a homolog of the upper vagina. Mesenchyme in this tissue differentiates into the peripheral zone of the prostate, under the influence of **dihydrotestosterone (DHT)**. In the presence of a functional fetal testis, DHT is produced locally from testosterone by the enzyme 5α-reductase. The more central tissue in this area, which may be of Wolffian derivation, forms the central and transition zones of the prostate. Cancers of the prostate are most likely to arise from the peripheral zone (Chapter 41).

External genitalia

Like the primordial gonads, the anlagen of the external genitalia are bipotential. In the 8th embryonic (10th menstrual) week, a urogenital slit, a genital tubercle, two lateral genital folds and two labioscrotal swellings become apparent as precursors to the external genitalia (Fig. 6.2).

While differentiation of the internal Wolffian duct system is testosterone dependent, the primordial external genital structures require the presence of DHT to differentiate into recognizably male structures. The source of the DHT is testicular testosterone, converted locally to DHT in the primordial external genitalia. In the presence of DHT, the lobes of the prostate gland grow out from the seminal colliculus where the urethra is developing from the bladder. The genital folds fuse to form the **penis** around the elongating urethra. The labioscrotal swellings enlarge and fuse to form the **scrotum**.

Descent of the testes from the abdomen into the scrotum is an androgen-dependent event during which the testes are pulled downward by a fibrous cord anchored to the developing scrotum – the **gubernaculum**. During development, a peritoneal fold around the Wolffian and Müllerian ducts (destined to eventually become the

tunica vaginalis) connects to the genital swelling, and the gubernaculum forms as a ridge under the peritoneum. The gubernaculum connecting the testis to the genital swelling does not grow as rapidly as the remainder of the embryo and hence each testis is progressively pulled down toward the developing scrotum. The testes sit just above the inguinal ring until the last 3 months of pregnancy, at which time they complete their descent through the inguinal canal into the scrotum. After full descent of the testes, the inguinal canal narrows, thereby preventing abdominal contents from herniating into the scrotum. Unlike differentiation of the external and internal genitalia that relies on placental hCG stimulation of testicular androgen production, testicular descent requires fetal gonadotropins. Disruptions in the fetal hypothalamic–pituitary–testicular axis result in failure of the testes to descend properly (cryptorchidism).

In the female, the folds of the urogenital slit remain open. The posterior aspect of the urogenital sinus forms the **lower two-thirds of the vagina** and the anterior aspect forms the urethra. The lateral genital folds form the **labia minora** and the labioscrotal swellings form the **labia majora**. The **clitoris** forms above the urethra. The gubernaculum that forms between the edge of the Müllerian duct and the ovary becomes secondarily attached to the cornua of the uterus as it differentiates. The gubernaculum in the female becomes the ovarian and round ligaments. Female phenotypic differentiation occurs in the absence of androgen and is not dependent on an ovary.

Exposure to specific androgens beginning in the 5th embryonic (7th menstrual) week of pregnancy is critical to the development of a recognizable newborn male phenotype. Fetuses exposed to endogenous or exogenous DHT at this time will undergo male differentiation, regardless of the genetic or gonadal sex. Lack of androgen activity will result in a female phenotype.

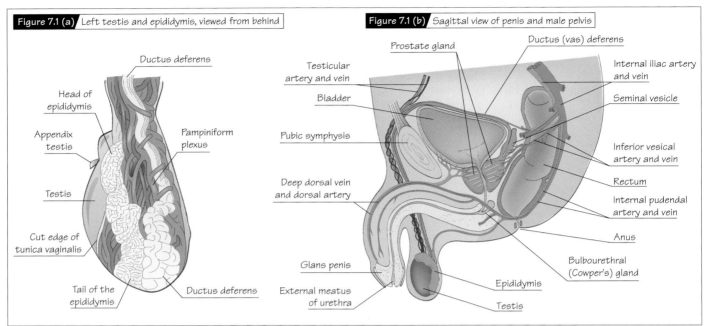

Figure 7.1 (a) Left testis and epididymis, viewed from behind

Ductus deferens
Head of epididymis
Appendix testis
Pampiniform plexus
Testis
Cut edge of tunica vaginalis
Tail of the epididymis
Ductus deferens

Figure 7.1 (b) Sagittal view of penis and male pelvis

Prostate gland
Ductus (vas) deferens
Testicular artery and vein
Internal iliac artery and vein
Bladder
Seminal vesicle
Pubic symphysis
Inferior vesical artery and vein
Deep dorsal vein and dorsal artery
Rectum
Internal pudendal artery and vein
Anus
Glans penis
Bulbourethral (Cowper's) gland
Epididymis
External meatus of urethra
Testis

Testes and epididymis

The **testes** are a pair of oval, slightly flattened bodies measuring about 4 cm in length and 2.5 cm in diameter. Together with the epididymides, they lie in the scrotum, an extra-abdominal sac just below the penis. The walls of the cavity in which the testes and epididymis reside are known as the **tunica vaginalis**. The tunica vaginalis forms from intra-abdominal peritoneum that migrates into the primitive scrotum during development of the male internal genitalia. After migration of the testis into the scrotum, the channel down which the testis has moved (processus vaginalis) is obliterated.

The **epididymis** is a comma-shaped structure that clasps the posterolateral margin of the testis. It is formed from the duct of the epididymis, an irregularly twisted tube. The epididymal duct is about 600 cm long. It begins at the top of the testis as the head of the epididymis. After an extraordinarily tortuous course it ends as the tail of the epididymis, then becomes the vas deferens (Fig. 7.1).

The testicular arteries supply blood to the testes and epididymides. These arteries arise from the aorta just below the renal arteries. The testicular arteries end in a dense vascular plexus, the **pampiniform plexus**, which courses just under the tunica vaginalis surrounding the testes. The plexus drains into the testicular veins. The pampiniform plexus dissipates heat out of the scrotum by vasodilatation and thereby has an important role in temperature regulation of the testes. **Like the ovarian veins, the right testicular vein empties into the inferior vena cava, and the left testicular vein into the left renal vein**. Lymphatic drainage of the testes is to the para-aortic nodes.

All the blood and lymph vessels to the testis and epididymis are bundled in a structure known as the **spermatic cord**. This structure also contains the **vas deferens** and any remnants of the processus vaginalis. The spermatic cord enters the scrotum from the abdomen through the inguinal canal.

The testis is the site of spermatogenesis and sex steroid production in the male. The epididymis is the site of final sperm maturation. The scrotum is basically a specialized dermal pouch that protects the testis and epididymis from physical injury and aids in heat regulation of the testes. Spermatozoa are very heat sensitive. Because the testes and epididymides are outside the body cavity, intratesticular temperature is typically lower than in the abdomen. Disorders of urogenital development that result in testicular retention within the abdominal cavity or inguinal canal can have dramatic effects on future fertility and increase the risk for testicular tumors (relative risk 3–8). Most of these are seminomas (Chapter 40).

Vas (ductus) deferens and seminal vesicles

The vas deferens is a direct continuation of the epididymis. It is a 45-cm-long structure that begins at the lower end of the epididymis and ascends along the posterior aspect of the testis in loose coils. After leaving the back of the testis, the vas deferens traverses the spermatic cord into the abdomen. The vas deferens may be felt as a firm hard cord on the posterior aspect of the spermatic cord as it traverses the scrotum toward the superficial inguinal ring. After crossing into the abdomen, the vas deferens curves medially across the external iliac artery toward the pelvis. From there, it crosses the obturator nerve and vessels and the vesicular vessels. The vas deferens then crosses over the ureter to meet the duct of the seminal vesicle. Together, the vas deferens and the duct of the seminal vesicle form the **ejaculatory duct** that opens into the prostatic portion of the urethra. The ejaculatory duct is short (2.5 cm) and lies very close to its companion contralateral duct as they pass forward through the prostate.

The **seminal vesicles** are a pair of hollow, sacculated structures located at the base of the bladder in front of the rectum. Each vesicle is about 5 cm long and more intimately connected to the bladder than to the rectum. During embryonic development, the seminal vesicles form as diverticula of the vas deferens. The structures share common blood and lymphatic supplies.

The Reproductive System at a Glance, Fourth Edition. Linda J. Heffner and Danny J. Schust.

Blood supply to the vas deferens and seminal vesicles is mainly from the inferior vesicular artery. The artery accompanies the vas deferens into the scrotum where it anastomoses with the testicular artery. Lymphatic drainage is to the internal and external iliac nodes.

The vas deferens functions in sperm transport. The seminal vesicles produce approximately 50–60% of the volume of the seminal fluid. Important seminal vesicle-derived semen components include fructose and prostaglandins.

Prostate gland

The prostate is a partly glandular, partly muscular organ that surrounds the beginning of the male urethra, firmly affixed by a connective tissue sheath just behind the symphysis pubis. The organ is about $2.5 \times 3.5 \times 4.5$ cm. The median lobe of the prostate, histologically referred to as the transition zone, is wedge-shaped, directly surrounds the urethra and separates it from the ejaculatory ducts. When hypertrophied, the median lobe may obstruct the flow of urine. Median lobe hypertrophy occurs commonly in elderly men.

The anterior prostate is composed mostly of fibromuscular tissue. The glandular tissue of the prostate is situated at the sides of the urethra and immediately posterior to it. This glandular tissue is subdivided into a central and peripheral zone based on embryology (Chapter 6) and histology (Chapter 8). The peripheral zone is much larger than the central zone and composed of about 50 incompletely defined lobules. Each lobule contains minute ducts that empty directly into the urethra just above the ejaculatory ducts.

The blood supply to the prostate gland is variable, but most commonly arises from the common origin of the internal pudendal and inferior gluteal arteries off the internal iliac (hypogastric) arteries. The veins draining the prostate are wide and thin-walled, forming a plexus that communicates with the plexus draining the bladder. Both drain into the internal iliac veins. The prostatic plexus also communicates with the vertebral venous plexuses; therefore, a tumor in the prostate may give rise to secondary growth in the vertebral column. Lymphatic drainage of the prostate follows that of the seminal vesicles and bladder neck into the iliac chain of nodes.

All the muscular tissues in the vas deferens, prostate, prostatic urethra and seminal vesicles are involved in ejaculation. Prostate secretions contribute ~15% of the volume of the seminal fluid. Important prostate-derived components include acid phosphatases, zinc, citrate and proteases that aid in semen liquefaction. Liquefaction enables sperm to escape the very viscous initial ejaculate.

Penis

The penis is composed chiefly of cavernous (erectile) tissue and is traversed by the urethra. The posterior surface of the flaccid penis is nearest the urethra and the opposite, more extensive surface is dorsal (Fig. 7.2). Most of the erectile tissue of the penis is arranged in three

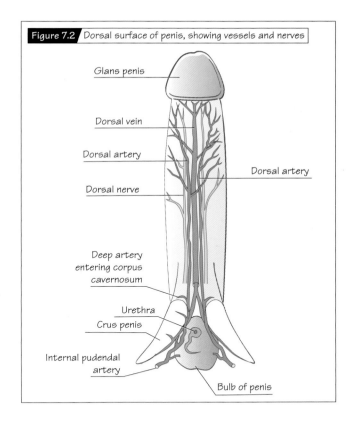

Figure 7.2 Dorsal surface of penis, showing vessels and nerves

Glans penis

Dorsal vein

Dorsal artery

Dorsal nerve

Dorsal artery

Deep artery entering corpus cavernosum

Urethra

Crus penis

Internal pudendal artery

Bulb of penis

longitudinal columns: the paired **corpora cavernosa** and the single median **corpus spongiosum**. The tip of the penis is called the **glans**. The glans of the penis also contains erectile tissue and is continuous with the corpus spongiosum. The glans is covered with a retractable folded layer of thin skin, called the prepuce or foreskin. Although it is not typically indicated medically, the operation of circumcision removes the foreskin and is still widely practiced in some societies.

The internal pudendal arteries supply blood to the penis, entering the organ on its dorsal surface and penetrating deeply into the erectile tissue of the corpora cavernosa. Veins draining the penis enter the prostatic plexus either directly or through the dorsal vein of the penis. Erection of the penis occurs when the extensive cavernous spaces of the corpora cavernosa and corpus spongiosum fill with blood. Engorgement of the penis inhibits venous return and allows maintenance of erection.

Innervation of the penis is critical for its erection. Penile nerve supply is derived from the pudendal nerve (2nd, 3rd, 4th sacral nerves) and from the pelvic autonomic plexuses. The lymphatic drainage of the penis is into the medial group of superficial inguinal lymph nodes.

The function of the penis is penetration. Penetration of the vagina of the female allows deposition of semen near the uterine cervix.

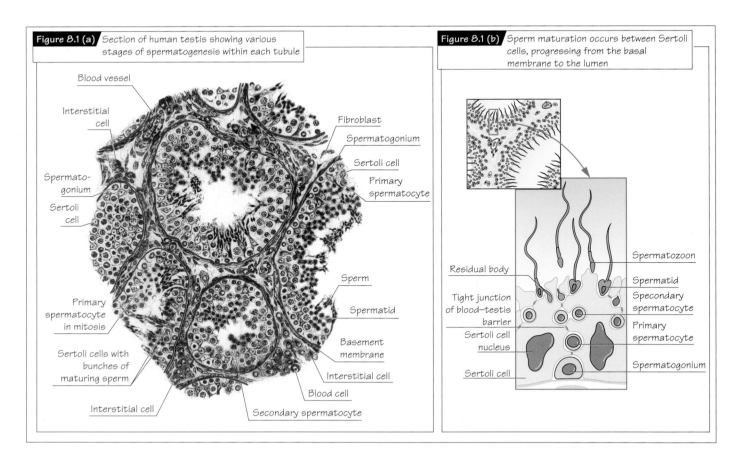

Figure 8.1 (a) Section of human testis showing various stages of spermatogenesis within each tubule

Blood vessel
Interstitial cell
Spermato-gonium
Sertoli cell
Primary spermatocyte in mitosis
Sertoli cells with bunches of maturing sperm
Interstitial cell

Fibroblast
Spermatogonium
Sertoli cell
Primary spermatocyte
Sperm
Spermatid
Basement membrane
Interstitial cell
Blood cell
Secondary spermatocyte

Figure 8.1 (b) Sperm maturation occurs between Sertoli cells, progressing from the basal membrane to the lumen

Residual body
Tight junction of blood–testis barrier
Sertoli cell nucleus
Sertoli cell

Spermatozoon
Spermatid
Specondary spermatocyte
Primary spermatocyte
Spermatogonium

Testes

The testes have two distinct functions: spermatogenesis and androgen production. Spermatogenesis occurs within distinct structures called **seminiferous tubules** (Fig. 8.1). These tubules lie coiled within lobules whose ducts all exit the testis into the epididymis. Androgen production occurs within pockets of specialized cells that lie in the interstitium between the tubules.

The seminiferous tubules are surrounded by a basement membrane. Juxtaposed to the medial side of this basement membrane are the progenitor cells for sperm production. The epithelium containing the developing spermatozoa that line the tubules is known as the **seminiferous epithelium** or **germinal epithelium**. In a cross-section of the testis, spermatocytes within a given tubule are in varying stages of maturation. Mixed among the spermatocytes are **Sertoli cells**. These are the only nongerminal cells in the seminiferous epithelium. Sertoli cells were aptly called "nurse cells" when first described by Sertoli in 1865. They are responsible for the metabolic and structural support of the developing spermatozoa. All Sertoli cells make contact with the basement membrane at one pole and surround the developing spermatozoa at the other. Sertoli cells have large, complex cytoplasmic "fingers" that extend around many spermatozoa at one time.

A wide variety of substances that are normally present in the circulation are excluded from the fluid within the seminiferous tubule. This phenomenon is similar to that seen in the brain as the result of the blood–brain barrier. The male reproductive system displays its own **blood–testis barrier**. This barrier allows the testis to be one of very few immune-privileged sites in the human body. While the function of this barrier is incompletely described, its ultrastructural basis is known to be the tight junctions that form between adjacent Sertoli cells. The barriers created by these tight junctions divide the germinal epithelium into basal and luminal compartments. The basement compartment contains the spermatogonia and the adluminal compartment, the maturing germinal cells.

Spermatogenesis can be divided into three phases: (i) mitotic proliferation to produce large numbers of cells; (ii) meiotic division to produce genetic diversity; and (iii) maturation. The latter involves extensive cellular morphologic remodeling aimed at facilitating sperm transit to, and penetration of, the oocyte in the female tract. Primitive spermatogonial stem cells remain dormant in the testis until puberty. At puberty, they are activated and maintained in rounds of mitoses at the basement membrane of the seminiferous tubule. From this reservoir of self-regenerating stem cells emerges several subtypes of spermatogonial clones until, after the final division, they exit mitosis as primary spermatocytes. Primary spermatocytes then undergo two meiotic cell divisions. These important divisions halve the number of chromosomes in the daughter cells. Cells undergoing the first of these meiotic divisions have very characteristic differences in their nuclear morphology that has led to a specific nomenclature (resting, leptotene,

The Reproductive System at a Glance, Fourth Edition. Linda J. Heffner and Danny J. Schust.

zygote, pachytene and diplotene; Chapter 4). The first meiotic division produces secondary spermatocytes (II) and the second, early haploid spermatids. The spermatids then undergo remarkable cytoplasmic remodeling, during which a tail, mitochondrial midpiece and acrosome all develop. Almost all of the spermatid cytoplasm is expelled as residual bodies during this remodeling; only a small droplet of cytoplasm remains within the head of the mature spermatozoon. The surrounding Sertoli cells phagocytose the residual bodies, a process that may transmit information about the developing sperm cell to the Sertoli cell.

Development of the spermatozoa within the seminiferous epithelium is a complex and highly ordered sequence of events in most mammalian species. In humans, the process appears somewhat less orderly, but still follows the general principles found in other species. In each, the number of mitotic divisions the spermatogonia undergo is fixed. In humans, four mitotic divisions occur. The length of time for an early spermatogonium to develop into a spermatozoon ready to enter the epididymis is also fixed and species-specific. In humans, it takes 64 ± 4 days for this process. As the spermatocytes move through the maturation process, they also move in waves toward the lumen of the seminiferous tubule.

The Sertoli cells enveloping the developing spermatozoa are homologs of the granulosa cells in the ovary. Sertoli cells phagocytose the extruded spermatid cytoplasm. They also function in aromatization of androgen precursors to estrogen, a product that exerts local feedback regulation on the androgen-producing (Leydig) cells. Sertoli cells also produce androgen-binding proteins.

Leydig cells perform the other major function of the testes – androgen production. The Leydig cells are homologous with the theca cells of the ovary. They produce large amounts of androgen from either circulating cholesterol or cholesterol made internally within their own smooth endoplasmic reticulum. Leydig cells are very large and, consistent with their intracellular activities, appear foamy by standard histologic assessment.

The most easily damaged cells in the testis are the spermatogonia. Irradiation, excessive alcohol intake, dietary deficiencies and local inflammation can rapidly induce degenerative changes in these cells. Excess heat also induces extensive spermatogonial cell degeneration but does not affect the length of the spermatogenic cycle.

Epididymis and vas (ductus) deferens

The ducts forming the epididymis and vas deferens have muscular coats composed of an inner layer of circularly directed fibers and an outer layer of longitudinally directed fibers. The muscle component of these structures is responsible for peristalsis that moves the spermatozoa along the ducts. The ducts are lined with a mixture of secretory and ciliated cells. The former aid in the generation of intratubal fluids; the latter assist in directed transit of intratubal fluids and cellular components.

Seminal vesicles

The alveoli of the seminal vesicles are lined with a pseudostratified epithelium whose cells contain numerous granules and clumps of yellow pigment. Some of the epithelial cells have flagella. The secretion of the seminal vesicles is a yellowish, viscous liquid containing globulin and fructose. This secretion provides the majority of the ejaculate volume.

Prostate gland

The tubuloalveolar glands of the prostate are lined with an epithelium that is highly responsive to androgens. The acini of the central glandular zone that surrounds the ejaculatory ducts are large and irregular. By contrast, the acini of the peripheral glandular zone are small and regular. These striking differences in glandular architecture, along with the observation that several unique enzymes present in the seminal vesicles are present in the central but not the peripheral glandular zone, suggests different embryologic tissue origins for these two parts of the prostate (Chapter 6). The epithelium of the prostatic tubuloalveolar glands produces the acid phosphatase and citric acid normally found in semen.

Penis

The erectile tissue of the penis is a vast, sponge-like system of irregular vascular spaces fed by the afferent arterioles and drained by the efferent venules. A pair of cylindrical bodies, the corpora cavernosa, is surrounded by a thick fibrous membrane called the tunica albuginea and separated by an incomplete fibrous septum. The veins draining the cavernous bodies lie just beneath the tunica. The interior of the cavernous bodies contains many partitions called trabeculae. Trabeculae are comprised of elastic fibers and smooth muscle embedded within thick bundles of collagen and covered by endothelial cells.

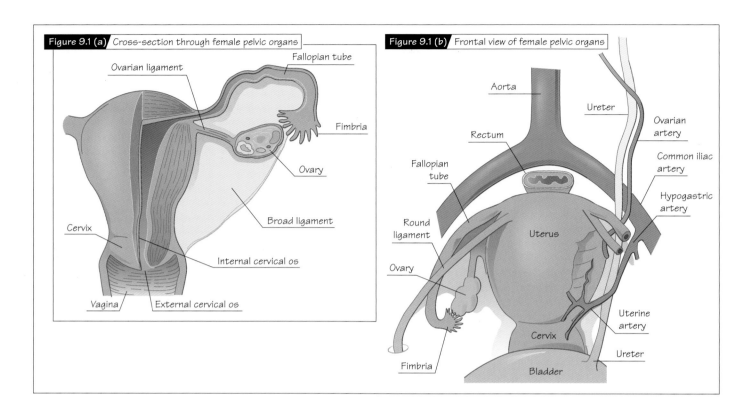

Figure 9.1 (a) Cross-section through female pelvic organs

Ovarian ligament
Fallopian tube
Fimbria
Ovary
Broad ligament
Cervix
Internal cervical os
Vagina
External cervical os

Figure 9.1 (b) Frontal view of female pelvic organs

Aorta
Ureter
Ovarian artery
Rectum
Common iliac artery
Fallopian tube
Hypogastric artery
Round ligament
Uterus
Ovary
Uterine artery
Cervix
Ureter
Fimbria
Bladder

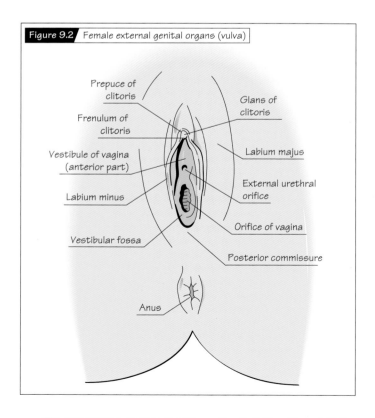

Figure 9.2 Female external genital organs (vulva)

Prepuce of clitoris
Glans of clitoris
Frenulum of clitoris
Vestibule of vagina (anterior part)
Labium majus
External urethral orifice
Labium minus
Orifice of vagina
Vestibular fossa
Posterior commissure
Anus

Ovaries

The ovaries are two small oval structures, each about $2 \times 4 \times 1.5$ cm, lying deep within the female pelvis just lateral to, and behind, the uterus. They are loosely attached to the uterus by a connective tissue band, the ovarian ligament (Fig. 9.1). To the practitioner performing a bimanual exam, they feel much like almonds sliding between the examiner's palpating fingers. After menopause, they may not be palpable at all.

The ovarian artery arises from the aorta just below the renal artery and is the ovary's major source of blood. The ovarian artery courses through the retroperitoneal space of the abdomen in close proximity to the ureter. Blood draining the ovaries traverses the ovarian veins. **The ovarian veins empty into the vena cava on the right and the renal vein on the left**. This anatomic difference in venous drainage is important; the more lateral position of the left ovarian vein makes it more susceptible to obstruction and thrombus formation, especially in pregnancy. The lymphatic drainage of the ovary feeds into the lumbar (para-aortic) nodes.

The functions of the ovaries are to produce mature ova for fertilization and to generate large quantities of steroid hormones.

Fallopian tubes

These are bilateral hollow structures that attach to the uterus at each cornua (corner). The fallopian tube is divided anatomically and functionally into three sections: the **cornua**, **isthmus** and **fimbria**. The cornual section is contained within the muscular wall of the uterus and

The Reproductive System at a Glance, Fourth Edition. Linda J. Heffner and Danny J. Schust.

provides a stable, strong connection with this organ. Fertilization occurs in the isthmus, a long, narrow, pencil-like portion of the fallopian tube. The fimbriated, or fluted, end of the tube is its most distal portion. The fimbria are finger-like distal projections of the fallopian tubes. They display continual sweeping-like activity and are known to reach into the cul-de-sac of the female pelvis to retrieve ovulated eggs that fall behind the uterus.

The fimbria of the fallopian tube are not enclosed within the parietal peritoneum of the broad ligament and hence communicate with the abdominal cavity. This anatomic connection creates the potential for foreign matter that enters the vagina (i.e., bacteria, sperm and chemicals) to gain access to the abdominal cavity by traversing the cervical canal, uterus and fallopian tube. This has important implications for exposure of the intraperitoneal cavity to carcinogens and for intraperitoneal spread of infections ascending through the reproductive tract (Chapters 42 and 46–48, respectively).

The blood supply to the fallopian tube is largely through the ovarian vessels, although anastomoses with ascending branches of the uterine artery occur within the broad ligament. The lymphatic drainage of the tube follows that of the ovary into the para-aortic nodes.

The functions of the fallopian tube include transporting sperm and eggs to the site of fertilization within the tube and returning the fertilized zygote to the uterine cavity for implantation.

Together with the ovaries, the fallopian tubes are covered with a layer of parietal peritoneum known as the **broad ligament**. This forms a double-thickness draping structure that is bounded superiorly by the round ligament of the uterus. The broad ligament connects the uterus, fallopian tubes and ovaries to the pelvic sidewall just lateral to these structures. It contains important blood vessels, including the uterine arteries and veins.

Uterus

The uterus is a single, pear-shaped, muscular structure that sits between the bladder and rectum in the female pelvis. A mature uterus weighs 30–40 g in a woman who has never delivered a baby and 75–100 g in one who has. It is anchored in the pelvis by three sets of connective tissue ligaments: the **round, cardinal** and **uterosacral ligaments**. The round ligaments attach to the cornua of the uterus anterior to the insertion of the fallopian tubes. These distinct cord-like structures traverse the pelvis, enter the inguinal rings bilaterally and attach firmly to the osteum of the pelvic bone. They provide some stability to the upper pole of the uterus but are not essential. The cardinal ligaments connect the uterus to the anterior abdominal wall at the level of the cervix. The uterosacral ligaments attach to the uterus posteriorly at the level of the cervix and connect to the sacral bones. The cardinal and uterosacral ligaments provide significant support to the female pelvic floor. Damage to these ligaments, including undue stretching from childbirth, can allow prolapse of the uterus and pelvic floor into the vagina or even through the vagina and onto the vulva.

The uterus is divided into three anatomically and functionally distinct areas: the **cervix**, the **lower uterine segment** and the uterine **corpus**. The cervix is composed largely of firm connective tissue and is typically about 4 cm long. About 2 cm of this protrudes into the vagina; the remainder is intraperitoneal. The cervix opens into the uterus via the internal os and into the vagina via the external os. The lower uterine segment includes the lower third of the uterus. The muscle of the lower segment draws the dilating cervix up and thins in labor. The corpus, the largest uterine segment, is composed of thick muscle. The very top of the uterus between the fallopian tubes is called the **fundus**, although this term is sometimes used to refer to the entire corpus of the uterus.

The blood supply of the uterus is complex. The fundus is supplied by vessels stemming from the ovarian arteries while the corpus, lower segment and cervix are supplied by the uterine arteries. The uterine artery is the largest branch of the anterior division of the internal iliac artery (also known as the hypogastric artery). The uterine artery travels from the pelvic sidewall to the uterus at the level of the internal cervical os and the cardinal and uterosacral ligaments. In doing so, the uterine artery crosses over the ureter, which courses directly from the kidney toward the bladder. This anatomic relationship must be considered during all pelvic surgery involving the uterus and its blood supply. Failure to remember that "water runs under the bridge" has caused many an avoidable ureteral injury.

The lymphatic drainage of the uterus follows its blood supply. The fundus and upper part of the body drain, like the ovaries, to lymph nodes in the para-aortic chain. The lower part of the body of the uterus and the cervix drain into nodes located along the internal and external iliac vessels.

The function of the uterus is to provide support for the growing fetus during pregnancy.

Vagina

The vagina is a tubular structure that spans the distance between its opening at the introitus of the perineum and the cervix. Its surface is covered with a compliant, rugated-appearing epithelium. The upper two-thirds of the vagina is most correctly considered part of the internal genitalia because of its embryologic relationship with the uterus. The hymen, which may remain as a thin transverse membrane through puberty or first sexual intercourse, is seen as an irregular circle of tissue at the opening of the vagina onto the vulva. The function of the vagina is to hold the penis during intercourse and to serve as a temporary receptacle for semen.

Vulva

The external female genitalia are collectively known as the vulva (Fig. 9.2). The vulva comprises the **lower one-third of the vagina**, the **clitoris** and the **labia**. The labia majora are the largest structures of the external female genitalia and surround the other organs, ending in the mons pubis. The mons pubis is a large fatty prominence that lies over the pubic symphysis. The mons and the labia majora are the only visible parts of the female external genitalia. One must part the labia majora to see the labia minora, clitoris and urethral opening. There are **numerous mucus-secreting glands** lining the vaginal opening. The largest and most important of these extend posterolaterally towards the buttocks and are called the Bartholin glands.

The internal pudendal artery supplies blood to the vulva; it derives from the posterior division of the internal iliac artery. The lymph drainage of the vulva is into the inguinal nodes.

The clitoris is the homolog of the penis and the organ of sexual arousal in the female. It is positioned just beneath the anterior fusion of the labia minora.

10 Microscopic anatomy of the female reproductive tract

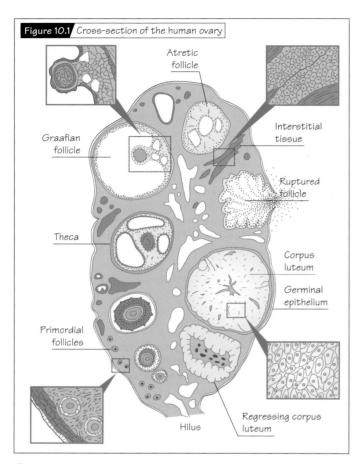

Figure 10.1 Cross-section of the human ovary

Labels:
- Atretic follicle
- Graafian follicle
- Interstitial tissue
- Ruptured follicle
- Theca
- Corpus luteum
- Germinal epithelium
- Primordial follicles
- Hilus
- Regressing corpus luteum

Ovary

The ovary has two distinct functions: germ cell production and steroid hormone biosynthesis. Germ cell support occurs in microscopic structures known as ovarian follicles. Resting follicles each contain a primitive or **primordial oocyte** surrounded by a single layer of cells, the **granulosa cells**. Surrounding the granulosa cells are a collar of cells known as **theca cells**. Theca cells produce androgens that are then converted to estrogens by the granulosa cells (Chapter 2). Steroid hormones produced by the ovary act within the follicle to support the developing oocyte and outside the ovary on target tissues.

The human ovary contains about 2 million oocytes at birth but only 100 000 at puberty. The number of oocytes continues to decrease throughout a woman's reproductive lifespan. This decrease occurs because mitosis of the primitive oogonia stops midway through fetal life and does not resume. At the time mitosis stops, the newly formed oocytes enter into the prophase of the first meiotic division. They will remain in meiotic prophase until either they are stimulated to mature for ovulation or they degenerate in a process called **atresia**.

The primordial follicles are scattered just beneath the connective tissue capsule covering the ovary (Fig. 10.1). This superficial position permits ovulation into the abdominal cavity. The earliest signs of follicular growth are: (i) an increase in size of the oocyte; (ii) a change in the shape of the surrounding granulosa cells from flat to cuboidal; (iii) an increase in granulosa cell number; and (iv) the appearance of

a **zona pellucida** around the oocyte. The zona pellucida is a sphere of gelatinous protein matrix immediately surrounding the oocyte. Once growth of the granulosa cells has produced three to four layers of cells, fluid begins to accumulate between the cells. This fluid resembles blood plasma and contains high concentrations of several protein and steroid hormones. When this follicular fluid accumulates around the oocyte, the follicle is known as a **Graafian follicle** and is approaching ovulation. Although as many as 20 follicles begin to mature in each wave of recruitment, typically only one successfully ovulates.

Ovulation involves expulsion of the egg through a thinned-out area known as the stigma. Stigmata can be seen with the naked eye as "blisters" on the surface of the ovary. Once the oocyte is released, the follicle collapses and the granulosa cells proliferate to fill the space left by the oocyte and its associated follicular fluid. They undergo transformation into plump, endocrinologically active cells known as lutein cells. These lutein cells produce a yellow pigment and the structure containing these cells is appropriately called the **corpus luteum**, or yellow body. During corpus luteum formation, blood vessels penetrate the follicular basement membrane.

Fallopian tube

The lumen of the fallopian tube is covered by a columnar epithelium with long **cilia** on the surface of many of the cells. The cilia constantly beat toward the uterus, a function that facilitates movement of the nonmotile zygote toward the uterine cavity for implantation. When cilia are injured or incapable of movement, an embryo may inappropriately implant within the fallopian tube itself (**ectopic pregnancy**).

Uterus

The vast majority of the uterine wall is composed of smooth muscle, called **myometrium**. The smooth muscle cells of the myometrium (myocytes) are attached by gap junctions, allowing rapid communication among neighboring cells and coordinated movement of the entire muscle mass. The uterus must be capable of enormous growth during pregnancy. This is accomplished by hypertrophy of the myocytes and by recruitment of new myocytes from stem cells residing within the myometrial connective tissue.

The cavity of the uterus is lined by a glandular epithelium, the **endometrium**. The endometrium is both an endocrine target organ and a gland. Under the influence of cyclic hormone production by the ovary, the endometrium undergoes striking microscopic changes in its glandular structure and function (Fig. 10.2). During the preovulatory phase of the menstrual cycle, the epithelial cells on the surface of the endometrium proliferate profusely under the influence of estrogen. The glands proliferate and elongate deep into the subepithelial layer known as the endometrial stroma. Small muscular arteries known as **spiral arteries** grow inward from the basal layer of the endometrium between the elongating glands. The hallmark of the **proliferative endometrium** is frequent mitoses in the epithelium. Immediately prior to ovulation, the endometrial glands are maximally elongated and markedly coiled.

With ovulation, the hormonal environment within the uterus becomes even more progesterone-dominant. In response to the change, mitosis ceases in the glandular epithelium and the cells form a single columnar layer within the glands. Within 2 days of ovulation, small

The Reproductive System at a Glance, Fourth Edition. Linda J. Heffner and Danny J. Schust.

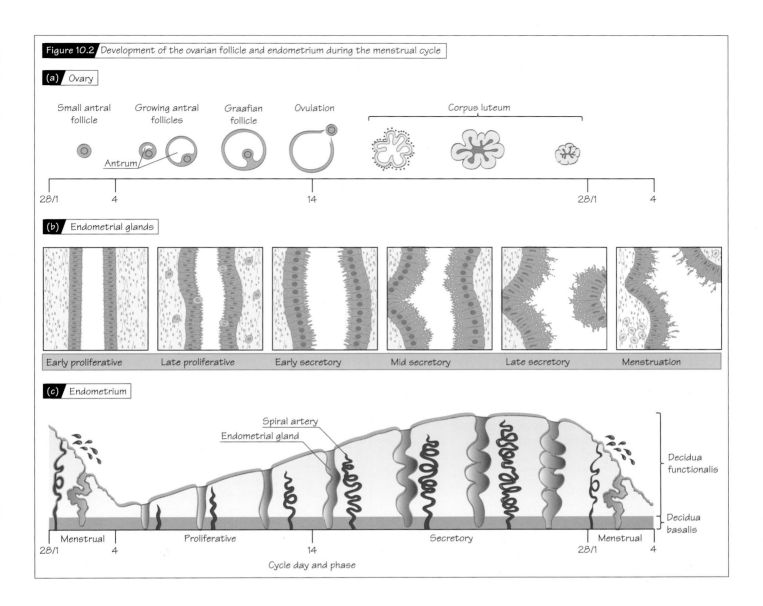

Figure 10.2 Development of the ovarian follicle and endometrium during the menstrual cycle

(a) Ovary

Small antral follicle | Growing antral follicles | Graafian follicle | Ovulation | Corpus luteum

Antrum

28/1   4   14   28/1   4

(b) Endometrial glands

Early proliferative | Late proliferative | Early secretory | Mid secretory | Late secretory | Menstruation

(c) Endometrium

Spiral artery
Endometrial gland

Decidua functionalis

Decidua basalis

Menstrual | Proliferative | Secretory | Menstrual
28/1   4   14   28/1   4

Cycle day and phase

subnuclear vacuoles form in the cytoplasm of the columnar cells. These secretory vacuoles are rich in glycogen and lipid and, by 4 days after ovulation, they migrate to the luminal side of the cells. Over the next 2 days, the vacuoles discharge their contents into the glandular lumens, leaving borders of the glandular cells frayed in appearance. This activity is the basis for the term **secretory endometrium**, which is used to describe the postovulatory endometrial changes.

Concurrent with these glandular changes are marked alterations in the endometrial stromal cells. With ovulation, stromal cells enlarge and acquire a foamy appearance indicative of increased metabolism. These cells become very eosinophilic and are known as decidual cells. **Decidualization** of the endometrium begins around the elongated and coiled spiral arteries. Decidualization then spreads under the surface epithelium and glands by 10 days after ovulation.

If implantation does not occur in a given menstrual cycle, progesterone production by the corpus luteum stops by day 13–14 postovulation. The endometrium undergoes ischemic necrosis and sloughs off, shed as menstrual debris. If pregnancy occurs, the extended lifespan

of the corpus luteum will prolong progesterone production and decidualization of the stroma continues. The endometrial stroma is an important source of several peptides in pregnancy, including prolactin, insulin-like growth factor binding protein 1 (IGFBP-1) and parathyroid hormone-related peptide (PTHrP).

The hormone-driven histologic changes in the endometrium are so predictable that they can be used to document ovulation and its timing.

Cervix and vagina

The cervix is composed largely of connective tissue. This is covered by a layer of mucus-secreting **glandular epithelium** inside the cervical canal (endocervix) and a stratified **squamous epithelium** on the portion of the cervix visible within the vagina (ectocervix). The transition between the glandular and squamous epithelium is known as the transformation zone. The **transformation zone** typically occurs very near the external os of the cervix. The zone is important in that it is a common site of dysplastic changes that can become malignant. The vagina is covered with squamous epithelium.

Figure 11.1 (a) Stages of genital development in boys

Stage	Description	Age at onset (years) Mean	Range
1	Preadolescent: Testes, scrotum and penis about the same size and proportion as in early childhood.		
2	Scrotum and testes have enlarged, texture of scrotal skin has changed. Testicular length >2.0cm <3.2cm.	11.6	9.5–13.8
3	Penis has grown primarily in length. Testes and scrotum growing. Testicular length >3.3cm <4.0cm.	12.9	10.8–14.9
4	Penis further enlarged in length and breadth. Glans develops. Further enlargement of testes and scrotum. Scrotal pigmentation darkening.	13.8	11.7–15.8
5	Genitalia adult size and shape. Testicular length >5cm	14.9	12.7–17.1

Figure 11.1 (b) Stages of pubic hair growth in boys

Stage	Description	Age at onset (years) Mean	Range
1	Preadolescent: No pubic hair (no thicker than over abdominal wall).		
2	Sparse growth of downy, long, slightly pigmented hair chiefly at base of penis.	13.4	11.2–15.6
3	Hair considerably darker, coarser and mostly curled. Hair spread sparsely on pubic junction.	13.9	11.9–16.0
4	Hair now adult in appearance but area covered still smaller than adult. No spread to medial surface of thighs.	14.4	12.2–16.5
5	Adult hair in appearance and quantity. Triangle is inverse of classical female pattern. Spread to medial surface of thighs but not above triangle base. In about 80% of men pubic hair eventually spreads further up beyond triangle base. This widespread pubic hair growth is not complete until the mid-twenties and may be called 'stage 6'.	15.2	13.0–17.3

Puberty is the process by which the immature individual will acquire the physical and behavioral attributes that allow him or her to reproduce. In males, puberty is largely the response of the body to the widespread actions of androgens. These are secreted by the newly awakened testes, under the influence of gonadotropins secreted by the anterior pituitary. While the progression of pubertal changes is predictable, the age of their onset differs dramatically in different areas of the world and even among children of different ethnic backgrounds within a particular region. Economic disparities may also be reflected in the age of onset.

Physical changes of puberty

In North America and Europe, puberty in males visibly begins with testes enlargement between ages 9 and 14. Secondary sexual characteristics progressively appear over the ensuing 2–2.5 years, and facial hair, the last to appear, will not be fully mature until 20–25 years.

The physical changes of male puberty have been divided into five stages using a system developed by Marshall and Tanner, who examined groups of English boys as they went through sexual maturation (Fig. 11.1). They then classified the relative and absolute changes in the sexual characteristics of the participants. Although they did not regard their findings as universal, their system has been widely used to describe the timing and progression of typical pubertal changes. Their descriptions must be recognized as specific to the demographics of their study population and to the years covered by the study. Patterns persist, but the characteristics and timing of these changes are affected by race, nutrition and other genetic and environmental factors.

Adrenarche

This describes the contribution of the adrenal gland to puberty. It is characterized by an increase in adrenal synthesis and secretion of the

The Reproductive System at a Glance, Fourth Edition. Linda J. Heffner and Danny J. Schust.

relatively weak androgens: androstenedione, dehydroepiandrosterone (DHEA) and dehydroepiandrosterone sulfate (DHEA-S). Although the adrenal gland contributes only 5% of the total circulating androgen pool in boys, these adrenal androgens are responsible for initiating axillary and pubic hair growth. They are converted in the periphery to the more potent androgens: testosterone and dihydrotestosterone (DHT). Testosterone and DHT then stimulate pubic and axillary hair growth as well as growth of, and secretion by, the axillary sebaceous glands. Axillary and pubic hair typically appear in parallel with increasing testicular size and visibly mark the onset of puberty.

The exact trigger for adrenarche is unknown. The best evidence indicates it is an intrinsic, programmed event within the adrenal gland independent of adrenocorticotropic hormone (ACTH). Adrenarche is distinct from pubarche and either may occur in the absence of its counterpart.

Testicular maturation

Testicular maturation at puberty involves initiation of androgen production by the Leydig cells, growth of the seminiferous tubules and initiation of spermatogenesis. The gonadotropins, follicle-stimulating hormone (FSH) and luteinizing hormone (LH) control all three events.

Throughout childhood, FSH and LH concentrations in both the pituitary gland and plasma are low. Pulse amplitude and frequency of both hormones are also low, suggesting that the gonadotropin-releasing hormone (GnRH) pulse generator is cycling slowly. This characteristic of the gonadotropin–pituitary axis has been called the juvenile pause. About a year before testicular enlargement occurs, the release of pulsatile FSH and LH begins to increase in both amplitude and concentration. When this begins, it is most notable during sleep. This marked diurnal rhythm in FSH and LH secretion is the first endocrinologic manifestation of puberty. While these diurnal variations may be striking during early and mid-puberty, they are almost obliterated by the end of puberty.

The initiation of puberty is thought to reflect the release of the hypothalamic GnRH pulse generator from CNS inhibition. The site and exact mechanism of this inhibitory release are unknown. While much evidence indicates that the source of the trigger also resides in the CNS, there is growing interest in the role of leptin, a hormone produced by fat cells, in the initiation and progression of puberty. Leptin has been shown to be one of the many factors that influence the maturation of the GnRH pulse generator. Individuals who lack the hypothalamic GnRH pulse generator do not undergo puberty (Kallmann syndrome; Chapter 29) and tumors or surgery in the region of the median basal hypothalamus can be linked with delayed or absent puberty.

The increase in size of the testes with onset of puberty is largely the result of increasing mass of the seminiferous tubules and initiation of spermatogenesis. Leydig cell stimulation results in a 10-fold increase in testosterone production over the course of puberty but accounts for only a small proportion of the change in testicular size. The Leydig cells occupy less than 10% of the total testicular mass.

Secondary sexual characteristics

Testosterone and its metabolites cause the following somatic changes in pubertal boys:
- Increased laryngeal size.
- Deepening of the voice.
- Increased bone mass.
- Increased mass and strength of skeletal muscle.
- Thickened skin.
- Increased and thickened hair on the trunk, pubis, axillae and face.

Somatic growth

Somatic growth at puberty is the result of a complex interaction between gonadal sex steroids, growth hormone (GH) and insulin-like growth factor 1 (IGF-1). Insulin and thyroxine are also necessary for optimal growth. The absence of GH, IGF-1 or IGF-1 receptor will lead to somatic dwarfism, even in the presence of normal plasma sex steroid concentrations.

Concomitant with the changes in the pulse frequency of LH that signal the beginning of puberty is a change in the amplitude of GH secretion. This appears to be the result of estrogen stimulation in both boys and girls. In boys, while the increase in GH can be initiated and maintained by testosterone, it does not occur with the administration of DHT. Further, GH secretion in the presence of testosterone can be blocked by the administration of tamoxifen, which blocks the estrogen receptor. In contrast, even miniscule doses of estrogen substantially increase GH concentrations. These findings suggest that the effect of testosterone on bone growth is indirect and probably secondary to aromatization of testosterone to estradiol. This is in stark contrast to the action of testosterone on muscle, where androgens act directly to increase muscle mass.

Bone growth occurs when testosterone, aromatized to estradiol, increases GH levels. This causes a parallel rise in IGF-1, a potent anabolic hormone that mediates many metabolic actions of GH, including trabecular bone formation. Normally, GH stimulates IGF-1 synthesis, and IGF-1 suppresses GH release in a negative feedback loop. At puberty, however, GH continues to rise despite high levels of circulating IGF-1. This allows for maximum linear bone growth during puberty. Outside of puberty, this combination of an increase in both GH and IGF-1 is seen only in acromegaly, a disease state characterized by autonomous GH secretion. Peak growth velocity in boys occurs when plasma testosterone levels reach 50% of adult male levels, and growth will continue until epiphyseal fusion occurs in the long bones. The sex steroids (perhaps via estrogen activity) are responsible for epiphyseal closure, which occurs at a median age of 21 in young men.

The determinants of final adult height are many and include genetic predisposition, body mass index at the onset of puberty, nutrition and length of puberty. Genetic determinants of bone growth appear to be carried on the distal short arm of the X chromosome. This locus does not appear to undergo X inactivation. Therefore, this locus, and any homologous loci on the Y chromosome, will direct final adult height. The effects of this genetic control pattern are apparent among men with the sex chromosome disorder Klinefelter syndrome; they have a 47XXY karyotype and are unusually tall, presumably because of the double dose of X-linked stature determinants.

Higher body mass indices in late childhood affect final height in both boys and girls. Children with increased body fat tend to enter puberty earlier. They begin their growth spurt after a shorter period of prepubertal growth and hence may not reach the full genetically predetermined adult height. Boys enter puberty later than girls and so have a longer period of prepubertal growth. Boys also experience a greater peak linear growth velocity during adolescence than girls. For both reasons, men tend to be taller than women.

Androgens have a direct anabolic effect on muscle mass. The increase in androgen secretion during puberty increases muscle mass in both boys and girls. Reflecting the higher levels of circulating androgens, this effect is more dramatic in boys.

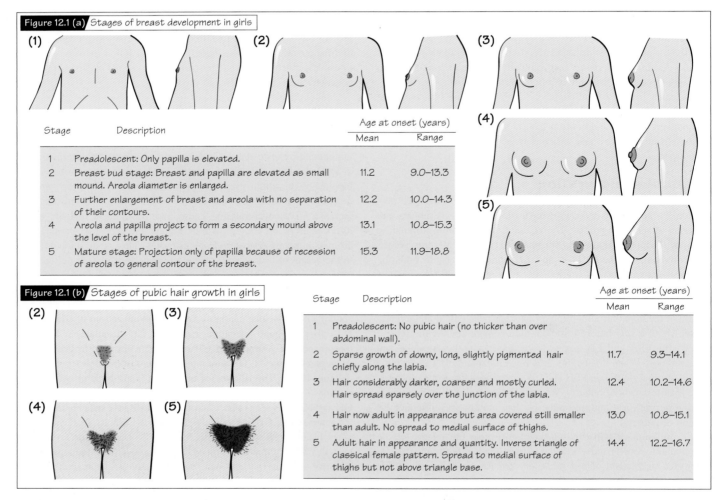

Figure 12.1 (a) Stages of breast development in girls

Stage	Description	Age at onset (years)	
		Mean	Range
1	Preadolescent: Only papilla is elevated.		
2	Breast bud stage: Breast and papilla are elevated as small mound. Areola diameter is enlarged.	11.2	9.0–13.3
3	Further enlargement of breast and areola with no separation of their contours.	12.2	10.0–14.3
4	Areola and papilla project to form a secondary mound above the level of the breast.	13.1	10.8–15.3
5	Mature stage: Projection only of papilla because of recession of areola to general contour of the breast.	15.3	11.9–18.8

Figure 12.1 (b) Stages of pubic hair growth in girls

Stage	Description	Age at onset (years)	
		Mean	Range
1	Preadolescent: No pubic hair (no thicker than over abdominal wall).		
2	Sparse growth of downy, long, slightly pigmented hair chiefly along the labia.	11.7	9.3–14.1
3	Hair considerably darker, coarser and mostly curled. Hair spread sparsely over the junction of the labia.	12.4	10.2–14.6
4	Hair now adult in appearance but area covered still smaller than adult. No spread to medial surface of thighs.	13.0	10.8–15.1
5	Adult hair in appearance and quantity. Inverse triangle of classical female pattern. Spread to medial surface of thighs but not above triangle base.	14.4	12.2–16.7

Puberty is the process by which the immature individual will acquire the physical and behavioral attributes that allow him or her to reproduce. In girls, puberty is largely the response of the body to the widespread actions of estrogens, secreted by the newly awakened plural-ovaries under the influence of gonadotropins secreted by the anterior pituitary. While the progression of pubertal changes is predictable, age of onset differs dramatically in different areas of the world and even among children of different ethnic backgrounds within a particular region. Economic disparities may also be reflected in the age of pubertal onset.

Physical changes of puberty

In North American and European girls, puberty visibly begins with breast development between the ages of 8 and 10. Other secondary sexual characteristics appear over the ensuing 2.5 years. Puberty culminates with onset of menstruation. The average age of menarche in Caucasian girls is 12.8 ± 1.2 years and, on average, 4–8 months earlier in African-American girls.

The physical changes of puberty in girls have been divided into five stages using a system developed by Marshall and Tanner, who examined groups of English girls as they went through sexual maturation (Fig. 12.1). They then classified the relative and absolute changes in the sexual characteristics of the participants. Although they did not regard their findings as universal, their system has been widely used to describe the timing and progression of typical pubertal changes. Their descriptions must be recognized as specific to the demographics of their study population and to the years covered by the study. Patterns persist, but the characteristics and timing of these changes are affected by race, nutrition and other genetic and environmental factors.

Adrenarche

This describes the contribution of the adrenal gland to puberty in both girls and boys. It is a developmentally programmed increase in adrenal synthesis and secretion of the weak androgens: androstenedione, dehydroepiandrosterone (DHEA) and dehydroepiandrosterone sulfate (DHEA-S). Adrenarche begins at about ages 6–8 years in girls. Secretion of weak adrenal androgens precedes the visible onset of puberty by about 2 years. DHEA and DHEA-S are responsible for initiating growth of pubic and axillary hair as well as growth of and secretion by axillary sebaceous glands. Axillary and pubic hair appear in parallel with the beginning of breast development and visibly mark the onset of puberty in girls.

The exact trigger for adrenarche is not known. It is independent of adenocorticotropic hormone (ACTH) release, gonadotropin release and

The Reproductive System at a Glance, Fourth Edition. Linda J. Heffner and Danny J. Schust.

32 © 2014 John Wiley & Sons, Ltd. Published 2014 by John Wiley & Sons, Ltd. Companion Website: www.ataglanceseries.com/reproduction

ovarian function, and appears to be an intrinsic, programmed event within the adrenal gland. Adrenarche is distinct from the other events of puberty (pubarche) and either may occur in the absence of its counterpart.

Breast development (thelarche)

The mammary gland, or breast, is an ectodermal derivative. The breast tissues are remarkably sensitive to hormones. Such hormonal effects are most notable during embryonic development and after puberty. The basic structure of the breast is common to all mammals although there exist wide variations in the number of mammary glands, their size, location and shape. Each mammary gland comprises lobulated masses of glandular tissue. Glandular tissues are embedded in adipose tissue and separated by fibrous connective tissues. Each of the lobes contains lobules of alveoli, blood vessels and lactiferous ducts. See Chapter 23 for a more detailed description of the structure and function of the human breast.

At birth, the breasts consist almost entirely of lactiferous ducts with few, if any, alveoli. These rudimentary mammary glands are capable of a small degree of secretory function ("witch's milk") within a few days of birth. Breast secretion in the neonatal period occurs in response to the high prolactin levels in the newborn infant following prior exposure of the fetal breast to high concentrations of placental estrogen during gestation. After placental estrogens are cleared from the neonatal circulation, the breast enters a dormant phase until puberty.

With the onset of puberty, ovarian estrogens induce growth of the lactiferous duct system. The ducts branch as they grow and their ends form into small, solid, spheroidal cell masses. These structures will form the lobular alveoli. The breast and alveoli enlarge. With menarche, cyclic estrogen and progesterone secretion begin and an extra phase of ductal and rudimentary lobular growth will occur. Adrenal corticosteroids further enhance duct development. The breasts continue to increase in size for some time after menarche due to deposition of fat and additional connective tissue. Final breast differentiation and growth will not occur until pregnancy.

Secondary sexual characteristics

Ovarian estrogens also produce the following changes in pubertal girls:
• Pubic hair.
• Keratinization (cornification) of the vaginal mucosa.
• Enlargement of labia minora and majora.
• Uterine enlargement.
• Increased fat deposition in hips and thighs.

Somatic growth

The pubertal growth spurt in girls typically begins 2 years before it begins in boys, accounting for about 50% of the 12 cm difference in average height between men and women. The other 50% results from a slower rate of growth during the spurt in girls compared with boys. The mechanisms by which sex steroids induce bone growth in girls are the same as in boys (Chapter 11). Structural growth ceases at a median age of 17 years in girls.

Menarche

The term used to describe the onset of menstrual cycles. It is the culmination of a complex sequence of events that involves maturation of the hypothalamic–pituitary–ovarian (HPO) axis to produce both mature ova and an endometrium that can support a zygote if fertilization should occur. The three stages of maturation of the HPO axis include: (i) an increase in the release of follicle-stimulating hormone

(FSH) and luteinizing hormone (LH) from the pituitary gland; (ii) ovarian recognition of, and response to these gonadotropins, allowing production of ovarian steroids (estrogen and progesterone); (iii) establishment of positive feedback regulation of the hypothalamus and pituitary gland by estrogens. The combination of these maturational events permits ovulation.

Throughout childhood, FSH and LH concentrations within the pituitary gland and plasma of boys and girls are low. As described in Chapter 11, the pulse amplitude and frequency of FSH and LH release are also low, suggesting the gonadotropin-releasing hormone (GnRH) pulse generator is cycling slowly. This characteristic pattern has been called the juvenile pause. The first endocrinologic manifestation of puberty is an increase in FSH and LH pulse amplitude. At its initiation, this increase is most notable during sleep, although the diurnal sleep–awake difference in FSH and LH secretion is almost obliterated by the end of puberty.

The initiation of puberty remains incompletely understood. Still, most agree it must be related to a release of the hypothalamic GnRH pulse generator from CNS inhibition.

There has been much interest in the observation that the age of menarche decreased by 2–3 months per decade during the 150 years preceding World War II and then stabilized over the next 50 years. A decrease was again noted in recent studies, thought to represent the influence of optimal nutrition. Onset of menarche is closely related to attainment of a crucial percentage of body fat. Two metabolic signals have been recently identified that can act centrally and may be causal in pubertal events: insulin-like growth factor 1 (IGF-1) and leptin. Serum IGF-1 levels increase during childhood and peak at puberty: the increase parallels that of DHEA-S, the marker of adrenarche. Leptin, a hormone signaling satiety, inhibits neuropeptide Y (NPY). NPY is a mediator of food intake, but also controls GnRH neuronal activity in the hypothalamus. Serum leptin levels increase in both sexes prior to onset of puberty. **Rising leptin levels inhibit NPY. This, in turn, releases GnRH from its prepubertal inhibition**. Leptin levels continue to rise throughout puberty among healthy females, but fall fairly rapidly after pubertal initiation in males.

Maturation of the ovary at puberty allows initiation of estrogen production by the granulosa cells surrounding the ova. Waves of granulosa cells undergo development and subsequent atresia as puberty progresses. Ova begin to mature under the influence of ovarian estrogen produced by these granulosa cells. In addition to oocyte maturation, estrogen from the granulosa cells will regulate production of gonadotropins by the pituitary gland. With complete maturation of the HPO axis, this estrogen will drive maturation of a dominant ovarian follicle, culminating in ovulation. With ovulation of the first ovum, the collapsing ovarian follicle reconfigures itself as a corpus luteum and begins to produce progesterone. The endometrium responds to estrogen by proliferating and to progesterone by converting to a secretory tissue capable of supporting embryo implantation. In the first years after menarche many menstrual cycles will be anovulatory, reflecting the incomplete maturation of the hypothalamic positive feedback response to ovarian estrogen. The menstrual bleeding patterns often encountered soon after menarche represent continuous exposure of the endometrium to estrogen and sloughing of proliferative or hyperplastic endometrium. Because no corpus luteum forms in the absence of ovulation, the endometrium cannot exhibit the progesterone effect that makes menstruation a self-limited phenomenon. This anovulatory bleeding can be very unpredictable and quite heavy. By 5 years after onset of menarche, 90% of girls have regular, ovulatory menstrual cycles.

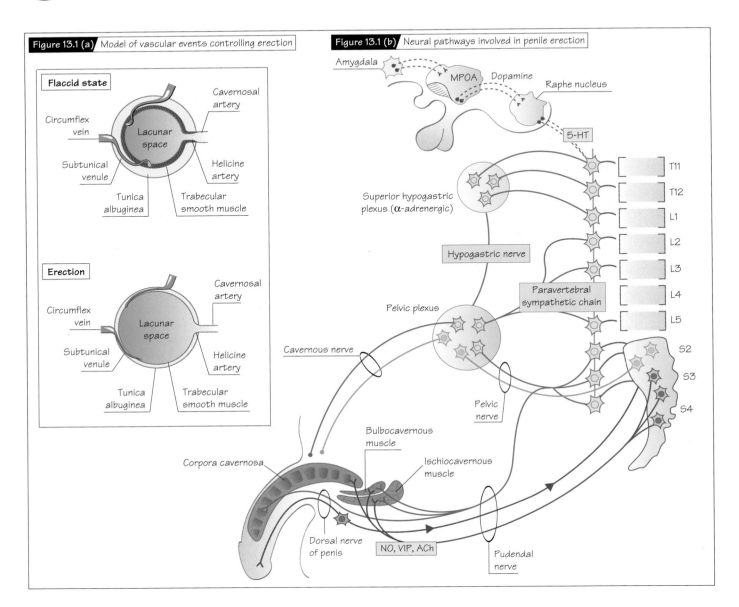

Figure 13.1 (a) Model of vascular events controlling erection

Figure 13.1 (b) Neural pathways involved in penile erection

Erection, emission and ejaculation

An **erection** is a complex neuropsychologic event. It occurs when blood rapidly flows into the penis and becomes trapped in its spongy chambers. The three systems directly involved in a penile erection are: (i) the spongy corpora cavernosa; (ii) the autonomic innervation of the penis; and (iii) the blood supply of the penis. Sensory, peripheral and central nervous system pathways integrate the response.

Although there are three erectile bodies within the penis, the two corpora cavernosa are primarily responsible for penile rigidity during an erection. The corpus spongiosum becomes tumescent during an erection, but does not become rigid. It serves to redistribute the intraurethral pressure so that the urethra remains patent and an effective conduit for the ejaculate.

The basic physiology of an erection is best understood if one considers each corpus cavernosum as if it were a single lacunar chamber

(Fig. 13.1a). Small (helicine) arteries transmit blood into the lacunar space, which is bounded by smooth muscle within the trabecular wall. These arteries have rigid, muscular walls. Exiting from the lacunar space are small venules that coalesce into larger (subtunical) venules. The subtunical venules drain through the tunica albuginea and form the emissary veins. Unlike arteries, veins have very flexible walls and are readily compressed.

When the penis is flaccid, the smooth muscle in the lacunar walls is in a contracted state. This contracted state is maintained by noradrenergic sympathetic fibers. Noradrenergic tone is blocked upon activation of the parasympathetic system and the intralacunar smooth muscle relaxes. Blood flows easily into the relaxed lacunar space through the helicine arteries. This distends the lacunar space and the subtunical venules and emissary veins are physically compressed by the expanded lacunae. In essence, the lacunar space becomes a large vascular "sink."

The Reproductive System at a Glance, Fourth Edition. Linda J. Heffner and Danny J. Schust.

Blood readily flows into this sink, but it is unable to exit via the penile venous system. Distension increases until the intralacunar pressure equals the mean arterial pressure.

Regulation of cavernosal smooth muscle is central to control of an erection. Simultaneous parasympathetic neural pathway activation and inhibition of sympathetic outflow are required for the smooth muscle relaxation that allows blood to flow into the sinusoidal spaces (Fig. 13.1b). The parasympathetic nervous innervation travels to the penis through the pelvic nerve whereas the sympathetic innervation travels in the hypogastric nerve. Numerous neurotransmitters are involved in the parasympathetic modulation of cavernosal smooth muscle relaxation. **Nitric oxide is the primary proerectile neurotransmitter**. It colocalizes with acetylcholine and vasoactive intestinal peptide (VIP) in nerve fibers terminating on the trabeculae of the corpora cavernosa and on the helicine arteries. Cavernosal smooth muscle contraction appears to be largely under α-noradrenergic control. Norepinephrine is the major antierectile agent.

Reflex erection can be elicited by afferent signals from sensory nerve endings on the glans; this reflex is mediated at the level of the spinal cord. The afferent limb of the reflex is carried by the internal pudendal nerves, which can also be activated by tactile stimulation of the perineum near the testes and scrotum. Erections can be modulated by supraspinal influences in the central nervous system. For instance, serotonergic pathways within the raphe nucleus of the midbrain can inhibit erections. The amygdala and the medial preoptic area of the hypothalamus appear to be important higher integrating centers in the modulation of erection. Dopamine is the candidate neurotransmitter in erectile control at this level.

The importance of testosterone in erectile function is not known. Nocturnal erections, which occur during episodes of rapid eye movement (REM) sleep, are testosterone dependent. In contrast, erections that occur in response to visual stimuli are not dependent on testosterone and will occur in hypogonadal men.

As ejaculation approaches, penile turgor increases even more. The smooth muscles in the prostate, vas deferens and seminal vesicles contract sequentially to expel the seminal plasma and spermatozoa **into the urethra** in a process known as **emission**. Emission is mediated by α-adrenergic sympathetic fibers that travel through the hypogastric nerve. Although emission and ejaculation are sometimes discussed as a single entity under the term ejaculation, these processes are distinct; ejaculation describes the ejection of semen **from the posterior urethra**. **Ejaculation** requires contraction of the smooth muscles of the urethra and the striated bulbocavernosus and ischiocavernosus muscles. These contractions are controlled through a spinal reflex mediated by the pudendal nerve and spinal nerves 2, 3 and 4 (Table 13.1).

Table 13.1 Erection, emission and ejaculation

Erection	Simultaneous parasympathetic activation and sympathetic inhibition
Emission	Sympathetic, α-adrenergic activation (hypogastric nerve)
Ejaculation	Spinal reflex (pudendal nerve; S2–4)

Hormonal control of spermatogenesis

Although ongoing spermatogenesis in the testes can be maintained qualitatively by testosterone alone, follicle-stimulating hormone (FSH) is required for initiation of spermatogenesis. The primary site of action of FSH within the seminiferous epithelium is in the Sertoli cells. FSH is delivered to the interstitial area of the testis via small arterioles. Once there, it diffuses through the basement membrane of the seminiferous tubules and binds to specific plasma membrane receptors on Sertoli cells. Activation of the FSH receptors results in the synthesis of both intracellular androgen receptors and androgen-binding protein (ABP). ABP is secreted from the Sertoli cells and binds androgens that have been produced by Leydig cells and diffused from their interstitial site of production into the seminiferous tubule. ABP transfers these androgens to the germ cells. Here, the androgens will be retained in the promeiotic germ cells that contain androgen receptors. Once FSH initiates spermatogenesis, the process will proceed as long as an adequate and uninterrupted supply of testosterone is available.

The FSH dependence of the Sertoli cells is analogous to the FSH control of the homologous granulosa cells in the ovary. Like follicular phase ovarian granulosa cells, Sertoli cells also secrete inhibin and activin. Inhibin, along with testosterone, inhibits pituitary FSH secretion in the male. Activin receptors have been identified on spermatogenic cells and may be involved in the FSH-mediated initiation of spermatogenesis.

Leydig cell function

Like the homologous theca cells in the ovary, Leydig cells respond to luteinizing hormone (LH) by synthesizing and secreting testosterone in a dose-dependent manner. In addition to LH receptors, receptors for prolactin and inhibin are found on Leydig cells. Both prolactin and inhibin facilitate the stimulatory activity of LH on testosterone production; neither can do this in isolation.

Regulation of gonadotropin secretion in males

The neuroendocrine mechanisms that regulate testicular function are fundamentally similar to those that regulate ovarian function. Hypothalamic gonadotropin-releasing hormone (GnRH), secreted in a pulsatile fashion into the pituitary portal system, acts on the pituitary of the male to stimulate synthesis and release of the gonadotropins, FSH and LH (Chapter 1). These two gonadotropins regulate the spermatogenic and endocrine activities of the testis. The male and female utilize the same negative feedback mechanisms to inhibit gonadotropin release by the pituitary. However, there is a major difference between regulation of the male and female hypothalamic–pituitary–gonadal systems. The postpubertal male has continuous gametogenesis and testosterone production while the postpubertal female has cyclic functions. The lack of cyclicity in males occurs because androgens do not exert a positive feedback on gonadotropin release.

Testosterone is the major regulator of LH secretion in the male. The negative feedback effect of testosterone is achieved largely by decreasing the frequency of the GnRH pulses released by the hypothalamus; although there are minor reductions in GnRH pulse amplitude. Testosterone also inhibits FSH release but its effects are not as pronounced as they are on LH. Combinations of testosterone and the Sertoli cell hormone inhibin are required to produce maximal FSH suppression.

14 The menstrual cycle

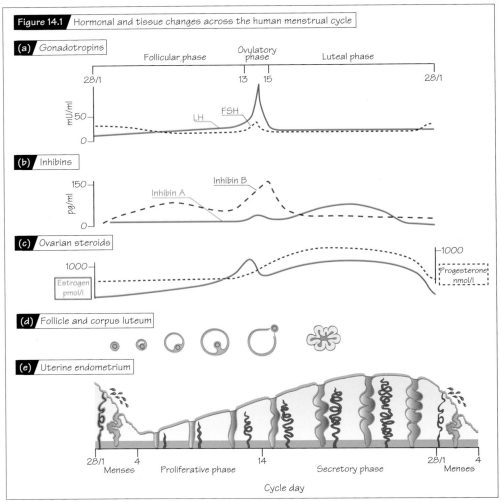

Figure 14.1 Hormonal and tissue changes across the human menstrual cycle

(a) Gonadotropins

(b) Inhibins

(c) Ovarian steroids

(d) Follicle and corpus luteum

(e) Uterine endometrium

Gametogenesis and steroidogenesis proceed in a continuous fashion in the postpubertal human male. In contrast, the postpubertal human female exhibits repetitive cyclic changes in the hypothalamic–pituitary–ovarian axis that allow: (i) the maturation and release of gametes from the ovary; and (ii) the development of a uterine environment prepared to support a pregnancy should fertilization occur. In the absence of conception, each cycle ends in menstrual bleeding. The pituitary gonadotropins, luteinizing hormone (LH) and follicle-stimulating hormone (FSH), link the hypothalamus and the ovary and mediate these cyclic changes.

The menstrual cycle is best understood if divided into the four phases of functional and morphologic changes in the ovary and endometrium: (i) follicular, (ii) ovulatory, (iii) luteal and (iv) menstrual (Fig. 14.1).

Follicular phase

Conventionally considered the first phase, this is the phase of the menstrual cycle leading up to ovulation. In a typical 28-day menstrual cycle, it comprises the first 14 days. In ovulatory cycles of more or less than 28 days' duration, the deviation from the average is largely caused by differences in the length of the follicular phase.

During this phase of the menstrual cycle, a cohort of ovarian follicles will rapidly mature, although only one typically becomes the dominant follicle, called the **Graafian follicle**. Those follicles that undergo final maturation in a given cycle have likely been growing for several months prior to that cycle. Progression from the primordial or resting state to the small antral stage is largely gonadotropin-independent. During the few days prior to the start of menstruation, a small cohort of these growing follicles, now at the small antral stage, is recruited for further gonadotropin-dependent growth. As one cycle ends, the scheduled demise of the corpus luteum results in a rapid decline in its hormonal secretion. The resultant fall in serum estradiol releases the central negative feedback inhibition on FSH secretion. Associated declines in progesterone and inhibin A are involved to a lesser degree. Increases in FSH secretion during the late luteal phase are accompanied by an increase in the pulse frequency of LH secretion.

Day 1 of menstrual bleeding is considered the first day of the follicular phase. During days 4–5 of this phase, development of the recruited ovarian follicle cohort is characterized by FSH-induced granulosa cell proliferation and aromatase activity. The theca cells of the developing follicle produce androgen precursors. These are converted into estradiol within neighboring granulosa cells. The process has been called the two-cell hypothesis (Chapter 2). Estradiol levels increase. The recruited follicles have several layers of granulosa cells surrounding their oocytes and a small accumulation of follicular fluid. FSH induces synthesis of

The Reproductive System at a Glance, Fourth Edition. Linda J. Heffner and Danny J. Schust.

additional FSH receptors on granulosa cells, expanding its own effects. FSH also stimulates synthesis of new LH receptors on the granulosa cells, thereby initiating LH responsiveness.

By days 5–7 of the menstrual cycle, a single, selected follicle predominates to the detriment of the others in the selected cohort, and will mature and ovulate between days 13 and 15. The predominant follicle is characterized by the highest mitotic index of all the recruited follicles, an optimal capacity for FSH retention in its follicular fluid, and high estradiol and inhibin B synthesis. Nondominant follicles have elevated androgen:estrogen ratios in their follicular fluid, suggesting suboptimal induction of aromatase activity, and will undergo **atresia**. Androgens appear to be key to the atresia process, as granulosa cells treated with androgen *in vitro* undergo apoptosis.

During the mid to late follicular phase, continued elevations in circulating estradiol and inhibin B suppress FSH secretion, so preventing new follicular recruitment. Continuous high elevations of circulating estradiol exert a somewhat unexpected effect on the pituitary gland; exponential increases in LH secretion. The ovary also exhibits increased responsiveness to the gonadotropins. Lastly, high estrogen levels cause growth of the endometrial tissue lining the uterus. These changes in the endometrium can be distinguished microscopically and are defined as the "proliferative phase" (Chapter 10).

Ovulatory phase

This phase of the menstrual cycle is characterized by a surge in pituitary LH secretion, culminating in extrusion of the mature ovum through the capsule of the ovary. In the 2–3 days preceding the onset of the LH surge, circulating estradiol and inhibin B rise rapidly and in parallel. Estradiol synthesis is at a maximum and no longer dependent on FSH. Progesterone begins to rise as the surging LH induces progesterone synthesis by the granulosa cells.

Key to ovulation is the midcycle positive feedback effect of estrogen on LH secretion. Proof that rising ovarian estrogens are central to ovulation lies in the observation that a gonadotropin surge can be elicited when prolonged elevated circulating estradiol concentrations are produced experimentally by 2–3 days of exogenous estrogen administration in women. The effects of elevated circulating estrogen are further augmented by the presence of ovarian progesterone. The site of the positive feedback actions of midcycle estrogen on LH secretion appears to be in both the hypothalamic neuroendocrine cells and the pituitary gonadotropes. The exact mechanism by which estrogen induces the midcycle LH surge is uncertain, but dopaminergic and β-endorphinergic neuronal modulation of the gonadotropin-releasing hormone (GnRH) pulse generator are involved. In fact, at midcycle, there is a 20-fold increase in sensitivity of the pituitary gonadotropes to GnRH. Further, the GnRH pulse generator can be inhibited by both synthetic and naturally occurring opioids, suggesting that opioids have a pivotal role in the neuronal control of the midcycle LH surge. A small rise in FSH occurs simultaneously with the pronounced rise in LH at midcycle, presumably in response to the GnRH signal.

Ovulation appears to require LH. The exact mechanism of this effect is unknown, although prostaglandins are thought to be at least one of the mediators. To this point, LH has been shown to stimulate prostaglandin biosynthesis by ovarian cells and inhibitors of prostaglandin synthesis inhibit ovulation in animals.

Luteal phase

After ovulation, the dominant morphologic and functional feature of the ovary is the formation and maintenance of the corpus luteum. In humans, the luteal cells make large amounts of estrogen and inhibin. In fact, the circulating estrogen concentrations during the luteal phase are in the preovulatory, positive feedback range. Characteristic of the luteal phase, however, are the uniquely high concentrations of progesterone and 17-hydroxyprogestrone secreted by the corpus luteum. Progesterone at these elevated levels prevents estrogen from stimulating another LH surge from the pituitary. Instead, in the presence of the combination of high concentrations of progesterone and estrogen, the preovulatory GnRH pulses are reduced in frequency, resulting in only baseline FSH and LH secretion.

The length of the luteal phase is more consistent than that of the follicular phase, normally 14 ± 2 days. If pregnancy does not ensue, the corpus luteum spontaneously regresses and follicular development proceeds for the next cycle. Only small amounts of LH are necessary to maintain the corpus luteum in a normal cycle. However, after 14 days, even basal LH secretion will not support the endocrine function of the gland. If pregnancy ensues, maintenance of the corpus luteum and progesterone production is critical to the success of the early gestation. Human chorionic gonadotropin (hCG) is a hormone homologous to LH. hCG is secreted by the placental tissues (trophoblast) of a developing pregnancy. Therefore, in the presence of pregnancy, hCG secreted by gestational trophoblast can maintain the corpus luteum until the trophoblast assumes the role of progesterone secretion (Chapter 18). High progesterone levels also create the "secretory phase" of the endometrium, which is marked by endometrial maturation that can allow implantation of the embryo (Chapter 16). The exact trigger for the demise of the corpus luteum in a cycle that does not result in pregnancy is unknown. DNA fragmentation patterns characteristic of apoptosis appear in the corpus luteum as early as the mid to late luteal phase.

The rise in FSH secretion near the end of the luteal phase is reliant on a concomitant drop in the high circulating levels of progesterone, estradiol and inhibin. It is clinically significant that an estrogen antagonist such as clomiphene citrate, administered in the luteal phase, causes a rise in circulating FSH levels and initiation of follicular recruitment.

Menstrual phase

The first day of menstruation marks the beginning of the next cycle. A new wave of follicles has been recruited and will progress toward maturation and, for one, ovulation. The phenomenon known as menstruation is largely an endometrial event, triggered by the loss of progesterone support from the corpus luteum in nonconception cycles.

Dramatic structural changes occur in the endometrium during menstruation, driven by complex and only partially understood mechanisms. Hormonally regulated matrix-degrading proteases and lysosomes appear to be involved. Matrix-degrading proteases are part of the metalloproteinase (MMP) family of enzymes whose substrates include collagen and other matrix proteins. Of the MMP family, seven members are expressed in cell- and menstrual cycle-specific patterns. Also, the endothelins, which are potent vasoconstrictors, appear to have maximum activity at the end of the luteal phase. Finally, the premenstrual fall in progesterone is associated with a decline in 15-hydroxyprostaglandin dehydrogenase activity. This results in an increase in the availability of prostaglandin $PGF_{2\alpha}$, a potent stimulator of myometrial contractility. Prostaglandin and thromboxane homeostasis direct myometrial and vascular contractions within the uterus. Control of such contractility is central to the creation of endometrial ischemia, the promotion of endometrial sloughing and the cessation of menstrual bleeding.

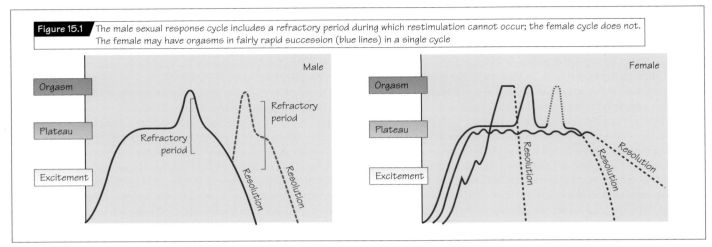

Figure 15.1 The male sexual response cycle includes a refractory period during which restimulation cannot occur; the female cycle does not. The female may have orgasms in fairly rapid succession (blue lines) in a single cycle

Successful reproduction is the ultimate definition of evolutionary fitness. Because fertilization occurs within the reproductive tract of humans, intimate contact between male and female is necessary for spontaneous conception to occur. Therefore, from an evolutionary view, human sexual behavior should ultimately be directed toward the physiology of coitus, which results in the deposition of sperm within the female reproductive tract. Of course, this purely procreational approach to sexual behavior is too simplistic. Humans differ from most animals, whose mating is seasonal and determined by hormonal cycles, in being sexually receptive regardless of fertility potential. Human sexuality is defined not only by procreation, but also by recreation and pleasure. The nonreproductive aspect of human sexuality is quite plastic and subject to individual and cultural influences. What is pleasurable to one individual may not be so to another. Normative behavior in one culture may be unacceptable in another. What does seem to be common to all human sexual responses is that both physiologic and psychologic satisfaction are central and motivating.

Most sexual encounters pass through five stages. The first stage, sexual attraction or arousal, was not included in initial descriptions of the human sexual response cycle. The latter four stages were first defined by the pioneering work of Masters and Johnson. Using hundreds of observations made during heterosexual interactions and masturbation, they divided the human sexual response into excitement, plateau, orgasm and resolution phases (Fig. 15.1). Although the validity of some of the data gathered by Masters and Johnson has been subject to question, their model remains the single best description of the physiologic aspects of the human sexual response.

Phases of the sexual response

Sexual attraction or arousal is the most individualized stage of the human sexual response. In many respects, sexual attraction and arousal are closely tied to personality. They are also the most culturally determined. For example, incest taboos forbidding marriage and intercourse between closely related family members are almost universal among cultures over time. In contrast, attention to women's breasts or weight in a sexual context varies tremendously among cultures. Interestingly, two variables of attractiveness do appear to be both universal and related to reproductive success: youth and health.

The nature of erotic stimuli can also be quite varied and include mental images, smells, sounds and physical events such as touching or stroking. If self-report and measurements of pelvic blood flow are used to indicate the level of arousal, men and women seem to be equally arousable. They differ dramatically, however, in the types of things that result in arousal. Novel or unpredictable situations and explicit visual stimuli, particularly body images, appeal to men more than women. Women generally prefer images with an emotional, romantic or familiar context. An individual's physical health and mental state contribute greatly to the threshold at which they can be aroused by a given stimulus.

During the next phase of the sexual response cycle, the physiologic **excitement phase**, sexual interest is stimulated by these psychologic or physiologic stimuli. This aroused state intensifies during the **plateau phase**. If stimulation is sufficient, **orgasm** or climax occurs. Orgasm is typically experienced as an explosive and pleasant release of sexual tension. Finally, during the **resolution phase**, sexual arousal dissipates. The physiologic changes associated with arousal and orgasm return to baseline. Although both men and women progress through the same phases of sexual response, they may differ in length and intensity in any given sexual encounter. The most notable physiologic difference between males and females is the presence of a refractory period in men. This is a part of the resolution phase following orgasm. During this period of time, sexual arousal cannot be restored and orgasm cannot occur in men. In contrast, sufficient stimulation can induce orgasm in women at any point during the resolution phase.

The basic physiologic responses of the human body to sexual stimulation are twofold. The primary reaction is **vascular congestion**. The secondary response is **generalized muscle tension** or myotonia. Reflexes activated within the spinal cord are modulated by the higher central nervous system and control each response.

Male sexual response

The human male's first physiologic response to effective sexual stimulation is penile erection. Erection occurs during the excitement phase, with vasodilatation of the lacunar smooth muscle of the penis leading to its engorgement and hardening (Chapter 13). Only a minimal degree

The Reproductive System at a Glance, Fourth Edition. Linda J. Heffner and Danny J. Schust.

38 © 2014 John Wiley & Sons, Ltd. Published 2014 by John Wiley & Sons, Ltd. Companion Website: www.ataglanceseries.com/reproduction

of sexual tension may accompany excitation and this phase of the sexual response can vary significantly in length.

Erectile stimuli may be either psychogenic or somatogenic. Psychogenic stimuli can include imagined sensory cues or direct visual cues, including explicitly erotic images. These signals are integrated within the limbic system of the brain and transmitted via descending projections to the spinal cord. They then travel via autonomic and visceral efferent nerves to the penis. Somatogenic stimuli include touching the penis or adjacent perineum. These tactile stimuli will reflexively activate the same efferents as the spinal cord pathway. This tactile reflex is typically preserved following spinal cord transection. The erection of the excitement phase may be quite susceptible to external signals and may resolve without progression. Changes in the physical surroundings, such as sudden loud noises, can impair penile erection in the excitation phase. Erection of the penis can also occur independent of the excitation phase of sexual arousal, observable in the newborn period and during sleep, especially in pubescent boys.

During the plateau phase, a minor involuntary increase in vasocongestion occurs and penile erection increases slightly. The size of the testes likewise increases and the scrotum and testes are drawn toward the perineum. There is a measurable rise in heart rate and systolic blood pressure. Just prior to ejaculation, a warm red rash may develop over the upper abdomen, trunk, neck and face. There is a diffuse and near maximal increase in muscular tension throughout the body. **Emission** immediately precedes ejaculation. During emission, muscular contractions are induced within the prostate gland, vas deferens and seminal vesicles and seminal plasma and spermatozoa are expelled into the posterior urethra. This process is mediated by sympathetic output traveling through the hypogastric plexus and can be abolished by α-adrenergic blockade. Once the plateau phase is reached, detumescence without ejaculation and orgasm is rare in healthy individuals.

During orgasm, somatic changes in the cardiovascular system are at their maximum, as is generalized muscle tension. Hyperventilation and vocalizations are common. Contraction of the smooth muscles of the urethra and the striated muscles of the bulbocavernosus and ischiocavernosus muscles expels the semen from the prostatic urethra. The pelvic floor and rectal sphincter may contract rhythmically. **Ejaculation** of the semen from the penis marks the height of orgasm. It is typically accompanied by release of sexual tension and an intense sense of pleasure.

Penile detumescence during the **resolution phase** of the male sexual response cycle occurs in two distinct stages. The primary stage of penile involution occurs very rapidly. The penis reduces in size from full erection to about 50% larger than its flaccid, unstimulated size. The penis is totally refractory to stimulation during this first stage. Secondary stage involution is a more extended process that returns the penis to its normal unstimulated size. The penis is only relatively refractory to stimulation during this stage. The penis progressively regains responsiveness. The excitement or plateau phase of the sexual cycle may be voluntarily extended by the male in an effort to delay ejaculation until his sexual partner is satisfied. This may be accompanied by a prolongation of the primary stage of detumescence after ejaculation.

Female sexual response
During the excitement phase of the sexual response cycle, somatogenic and psychogenic stimuli arouse the female through neural pathways similar to those described for the male. The clitoral response to arousal is less predictable than is that of its homolog, the penis. Tactile stimulation of the female perineum or the glans clitoris can elicit vasocongestion, engorgement of the body of the clitoris and erection, but only in some women. The response of the vagina during the excitement phase is much more predictable and consistent than that of the clitoris. Vaginal lubrication begins 10–30 s after receipt of arousing stimuli and continues progressively through orgasm. The more prolonged the excitement and plateau phases, the greater the production of vaginal lubrication. The upper two-thirds of the vagina also expand and lengthen during the excitement phase. This elevates the uterus into the false pelvis, repositions the cervix above the vaginal floor and "tents" the midvaginal plane. These changes result in an increase in the circumference of the vaginal diameter, largely at the level of the cervix. Finally, the labia minora become markedly engorged with blood during the excitement phase. The engorged labia minora displace the labia majora upward and outward away from the vaginal introitus. This increase in the diameter of the labia minora adds at least 1 cm to the functional length of the vagina.

During the plateau phase, the most striking change in the female genitalia is the florid coloration of the labia minora accompanying vascular congestion. This beet red appearance is the single most consistent physical marker for sexual arousal in the female. The clitoris retracts behind a tissue hood formed by the labia. The respiratory rate, heart rate and blood pressure all increase late in the plateau phase; the magnitude of these changes are not as marked in women as in men. Generalized myotonia may be present, including spastic contractions of the striated muscles of the hands and feet. The latter are referred to as carpopedal spasms.

During heterosexual coitus, penetration of the penis into the vagina can heighten a woman's sexual arousal by indirectly stimulating the retracted clitoris. This occurs because of traction on the engorged labia minora whose fused anterior segment forms the clitoral hood. The glans of the clitoris, however, is extremely sensitive in the aroused state. For this reason, direct and prolonged contact may be irritating.

Similar to the male, orgasm in the female involves rhythmic contractions of the muscles of the reproductive organs followed by physical release from the vasocongestive and myotonic tensions developed during arousal. Typically, orgasmic contractions begin in the lower third of the vagina and evolve to encompass the entire vagina and uterus. A sex flush, which can also include diffuse fine perspiration, may develop over the woman's entire body. The resolution phase of the sexual response cycle of women involves decongestion of the labia, detumescence of the clitoris if it has occurred, and relaxation of the vagina.

There are four major physiologic differences between male and female orgasms. First, emission and ejaculation do not occur in the female. Second, if sexual stimulation occurs before a woman drops below plateau phase levels of arousal, the female is capable of rapidly successive orgasms. Third, females more commonly reach the plateau phase, remain there for brief or prolonged periods of time but then return to the unstimulated state without orgasm than their male counterparts. Finally, the female orgasm may last for a relatively long period compared with that of the male.

16 Fertilization and the establishment of pregnancy

Figure 16.1 Key steps in fertilization, early embryogenesis and implantation

The egg

At ovulation, the egg is arrested in metaphase of the second meiotic division (Chapter 4). It is surrounded by a proteinaceous sphere called the **zona pellucida**. Those granulosa cells that adhered to the surface of the zona pellucida and were expelled with the egg from the ovary remain attached as the cumulus. Sperm that fertilize the egg must first negotiate these surrounding layers before they can penetrate the egg cell membrane. The oocyte will remain viable for at least 6–24 h once ovulated.

The sperm

With coitus, millions of sperm are deposited in the upper vagina. Most will never arrive at the site of fertilization. Abnormal sperm can rarely make this long trip successfully and even most of the healthy spermatozoa die along the way. The vast majority leak from the vagina upon liquification of the semen. Only a small proportion enters the cervix, where sperm will be found within minutes of coitus. Here they can survive within the epithelial crypts for hours. Sperm cannot traverse the cervix into the uterine cavity unless the cervical mucous is receptive. This typically occurs at midcycle when estrogen levels are high and progesterone is low. Estrogen softens the cervical stroma and makes cervical secretions thin and watery. Progesterone has opposite effects, a combination hostile to spermatozoa.

In the best of conditions, it takes 2–7 h for sperm to move through the uterus to the site of fertilization within the oviduct. Sperm transport results from self-propulsion, aided by the ciliary beating of cells within the uterine lining. Typically, only several hundred sperm reach the oviducts, where they will linger in a quiet state until ovulation occurs. After ovulation, these spermatozoa are reactivated and begin moving toward the egg. The signal that attracts the sperm to the egg is unknown. Human spermatozoa can survive for approximately of 24–48 h in the female reproductive tract.

Freshly ejaculated spermatozoa are not capable of fertilizing an egg. They acquire the ability to penetrate the cell layers surrounding the oocyte through a process known as **capacitation**. Although capacita-

The Reproductive System at a Glance, Fourth Edition. Linda J. Heffner and Danny J. Schust.

tion can be induced *in vitro* under the proper culture conditions, it occurs *in vivo* within the female reproductive tract. During capacitation, the glycoprotein coat that adheres to the spermatozoa cell membranes is initially removed, initiating changes in the surface charge of the sperm membrane and reorganization of that membrane. Capacitated sperm change their tail movements from regular undulating waves to whip-like, thrashing movements that propel the sperm forward. At the biochemical level, capacitated sperm acquire increased calcium sensitivity and elevated internal cAMP levels. Capacitation takes several hours both *in vivo* and *in vitro*.

Sperm capacitation allows for the **acrosome reaction**. In the absence of an acrosome reaction, a sperm is incapable of penetrating the zona pellucida. Contact of an intact, capacitated sperm with the zona pellucida of an egg allows interaction of a specific sperm cell surface glycoprotein, ZP3, with specific zona protein. These interactions are likely mediated by the sugars on sperm–egg binding proteins. ZP3-binding induces further calcium influx into the spermatozoa and intracellular cAMP levels rise. The acrosome swells, its outer membrane fuses with the sperm plasma membrane, and the enzymatic contents of the acrosome are released into the extracellular space surrounding the head of the sperm. This exposes the inner acrosomal membrane and another zona-binding protein, ZP2, to the oocyte zona. ZP2 binding holds sperm near the egg. Proteolytic enzymes released from the acrosome then facilitate penetration of the zona pellucida by the whiplashing sperm. Complete penetration of the zona takes about 15 minutes.

Fertilization

Penetration of the zona pellucida allows contact between spermatozoa and the oocyte membrane (Fig. 16.1). The germ cell membranes fuse almost immediately and the sperm cell stops moving. The sperm nucleus enters the egg cytoplasm.

Three important events are triggered within the oocyte by the rise in intracellular calcium that occurs in the oocyte upon fusion of sperm and egg cell membranes. The egg cell membrane depolarizes, preventing membrane fusion with additional spermatozoa. This is the **primary block to polyspermy**. It assures that only one male pronucleus is available for fusion with the female pronucleus and protects the diploid status of the zygote. The second event is known as the **cortical reaction**. Cortical granules lie just beneath the egg cell membrane, and with the cortical reaction they fuse with the membrane and release their contents into the zona pellucida. This hardens the zona and impairs the ability of sperm to bind to it – a **secondary block to polyspermy**. The third event involves resumption of the second meiotic division of the egg. The second polar body is formed and extruded from the egg, thereby assuring that the female pronucleus is haploid. Again, the diploid zygote is protected. Failure to preserve the diploid state of the conceptus is a frequent cause of early pregnancy failure (Chapter 36).

Upon entry into the egg, sperm cytoplasm mixes with that of the egg and the sperm nuclear membrane breaks down. A new membrane forms around the sperm chromatin, forming the **male pronucleus**. A new oocyte nuclear membrane also forms around the **female pronucleus**. DNA synthesis begins during this period as the haploid pronuclei prepare for the first mitotic division of the zygote. The pronuclear membranes break down, the parental chromosomes mix and the metaphase mitotic spindle forms. At about 24h after fertilization, the chromosomes separate and the first cell division occurs.

During the first few embryonic cell divisions, no new mRNA is synthesized from the nuclear DNA of the conceptus. The embryo stays the same total size and the size of each individual cell decreases accordingly. Thus, the early embryo uses only maternal cell components to develop and important signals must be transmitted to the embryo through the oocyte cytoplasm. These signals likely reside in **mitochondrial DNA**, which is replicated during early embryonic cell division. In fact, mitochondrial DNA is quite stable and can be traced through generations to determine maternal lineage.

Establishment of pregnancy

After fertilization, a successful pregnancy must implant within the wall of the uterus and inform the mother that pregnancy adaptations must occur. Without these two important events, the zygote will simply wash out of the uterus with the next menses.

The cleaving zygote floats in the oviduct for approximately 1 week, progressing from the 16-cell stage through the solid **morula** (mulberry) stage to the 32–64 cell **blastocyst stage**. The latter stage requires formation of the fluid-containing blastocyst cavity. The blastocyst contains two distinct differentiated embryonic cell types: the outer **trophectoderm** cells and the **inner cell mass**. The trophectoderm cells will eventually form the placenta. The inner cell mass will form the fetus and fetal membranes. It is at the blastocyst stage that the conceptus enters the uterus.

During the time that it spends in the oviduct, the conceptus remains surrounded by the zona pellucida. After about 2 days in the uterus, the blastocyst will lose or "hatch" from the zona pellucida. On hatching, the trophectodermal cells of the blastocyst differentiate into **trophoblast** cells. These simultaneous processes allow trophoblast cells to make direct contact with the uterine luminal epithelial cells. The blastocyst attaches to and invades the uterine lining. Within hours, the surface epithelium immediately underlying the conceptus becomes eroded and nearby cells lyse, releasing primary metabolic substrates used by the blastocyst. The endometrium undergoes dramatic biochemical and morphologic changes called **decidualization**, a process beginning at the point of attachment and spreading in a concentric wave from the point of implantation. The decidualized endometrium will heal over the conceptus so that the entire implantation becomes buried within the endometrium.

As the embryo invades maternal tissues the trophoblast cells further differentiate into two layers: inner **cytotrophoblast cells** and an outer **syncytiotrophoblast** (Chapter 17). The syncytiotrophoblast is a continuous, multinucleated layer that covers the interstitial space and arises from fusion of the underlying cytotrophoblast progenitor cells. Syncytiotrophoblast is active in placental hormone secretion and in nutrient transport from mother to fetus. A separate subset of cytotrophoblast cells acquires invasive properties and traverses endometrial stroma to reach maternal blood vessels, including the spiral arteries of the endometrium. Appropriate invasion and subsequent remodeling of the spiral arteries by these extravillous cytotrophoblast cells is key to a normal pregnancy outcome (Chapter 38).

A number of growth factors are integral to successful implantation: (i) leukemia inhibitory factor, a cytokine; (ii) the integrins, which mediate cell–cell interactions; and (iii) transforming growth factor beta (TGF-β), which stimulates syncytium formation and inhibits trophoblast invasion. Epidermal growth factor and interleukin 1β are also important mediators of invasion.

Implantation occurs about 7–10 days after ovulation. If the conceptus is to survive more than 14 days after ovulation, the ovarian corpus luteum must continue to secrete progesterone. **Human chorionic gonadotropin** (hCG) produced by the developing trophoblast and secreted into the maternal bloodstream acts like luteinizing hormone, supporting the corpus luteum by inhibiting luteal regression (Chapters 14 and 18).

17 Placental structure and function

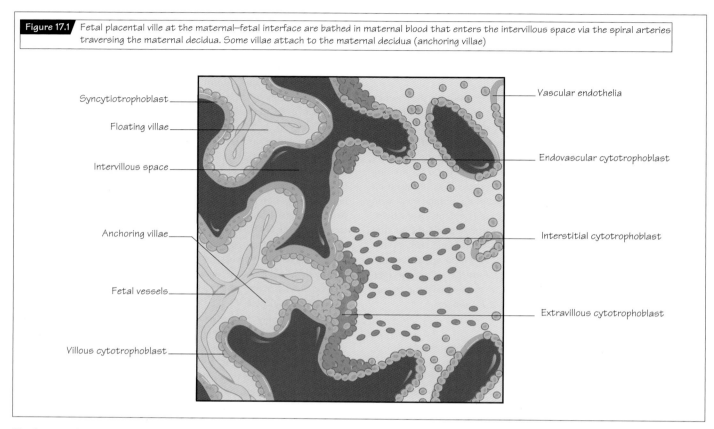

Figure 17.1 Fetal placental ville at the maternal–fetal interface are bathed in maternal blood that enters the intervillous space via the spiral arteries traversing the maternal decidua. Some villae attach to the maternal decidua (anchoring villae)

- Syncytiotrophoblast
- Floating villae
- Intervillous space
- Anchoring villae
- Fetal vessels
- Villous cytotrophoblast
- Vascular endothelia
- Endovascular cytotrophoblast
- Interstitial cytotrophoblast
- Extravillous cytotrophoblast

The human placenta is the sole interface between the mother and her developing embryo/fetus. Humans differ from most other mammals in that maternal blood comes into direct contact with fetally derived placental tissues. This organization characterizes the hemochorial placenta through which all maternal nutrients and fetal wastes must pass. The placenta is a very active organ that has specialized mechanisms to promote fetal growth and survival. These include, but are not limited to, efficient gas exchange, active transport of energy substrates, immunologic tolerance of the fetal allograft and fetal acquisition of maternal immunity.

Placental morphology

After it enters the uterus, the human blastocyst resides within the uterine cavity for 2–3 days prior to implantation into the decidualized uterine endometrium (Chapter 16). Implantation can be divided into three distinct processes: apposition of the blastocyst to the endometrial epithelium at the site of implantation, a brief period of stable adhesion of the blastocyst to this epithelium and invasion of the developing embryo into the uterine decidua. The signals governing these processes are complex and involve active maternal and fetal participation. **Apposition** requires the secretion of soluble mediators by uterine epithelia and the blastocyst that include interleukins, prostaglandins and leukemia inhibiting factor (LIF). **Adhesion** is promoted by the expression of ligands on the surface of the developing embryo that specifically bind to receptors expressed on the uterine lining at the site of implantation. One receptor–ligand pair that has been implicated in

embryo adhesion is heparin-binding epidermal growth factor and heparin sulfate proteoglycans. Also important in the adhesion process is a family of adhesion molecules expressed on uterine epithelia in a time-specific and hormone-dependent fashion: the integrins. **Invasion** of the blastocyst into the maternal uterine decidua requires an alteration in the expression of embryonic surface molecules, from those promoting adhesion to the endometrium to others that stimulate invasion of vascular structures. During invasion, the embryo also begins to secrete proteases that digest between the cells of the decidua and allow invasion to areas deep within the uterine lining.

The blastocyst is comprised of two populations of cells (see Fig. 16.1): one will become the fetus, the other, the placenta. At the blastocyst stage, the embryo is characterized by a fluid-filled cavity (the blastocele) surrounded by a layer of trophectoderm cells. The trophectoderm will develop into the placenta. Within the trophectoderm shell is a collection of cells called the inner cell mass. All nonplacental fetal tissues will arise from the inner cell mass.

During implantation, trophectoderm cells begin to differentiate into cellular subtypes that will characterize the mature placenta. The mature placenta is comprised of a mass of tree-like placental cotyledons called villae, which are bathed in maternal blood (Fig. 17.1). Blood enters the space between the villae through low-resistance, high-flow vessels that branch from the maternal uterine spiral arteries. Fetal vessels are located within the core of each placental cotyledon. Loose connective tissue and layers of trophoblast cells surround each fetal vessel. The inner layers of the trophoblast shell around the fetal

The Reproductive System at a Glance, Fourth Edition. Linda J. Heffner and Danny J. Schust.

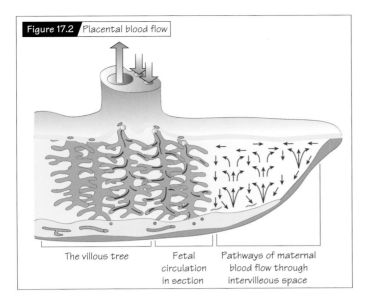

Figure 17.2 Placental blood flow

The villous tree | Fetal circulation in section | Pathways of maternal blood flow through intervilleous space

system. The fetal tissue, which contains both a maternal and paternal haplotype, is a hemi-allograph. Typically, when an immunocompetent organism encounters genetically foreign tissue, rejection occurs. This does not happen in pregnancy. Maternal immunologic tolerance to the fetal allograft remains incompletely understood. Alterations in maternal immune responsivity may occur because of the maternal reproductive hormones. Progesterone and prolactin have remarkable immunosuppressive activities and both are elevated in pregnancy. Also, the villous cytotrophoblast cells of the placenta do not express major histocompatability complex (MHC) class I and MHC class II transplantation antigens on their surfaces. Extravillous cytotrophoblast cells also lack MHC class II and classic MHC class I antigens but instead express a unique subset of nonclassic MHC class I products. These nonclassic products are thought to be important in interactions between placental cells and the very unique populations of immune cells residing at the site of implantation. Placental tissues may also have altered metabolic processes that promote immunosuppression. For instance, placental tissues rapidly degrade tryptophan, an amino acid that activates T lymphocytes.

vessels are comprised of **cytotrophoblast** cells. The outer layer of the placental villae is coated by a multinucleated syncytium of fused cytotrophoblast cells called the **syncytiotrophoblast**. The syncytiotrophoblast is directly bathed in maternal blood in the mature placenta.

The vast majority of placental cotyledons/villae float freely in the intervillous space. Here, they are surrounded by maternal blood. A subset of villae completely cross the intervillous space and attach to the maternal uterine decidua. These are called anchoring villae. At the maternal end of the anchoring villae, a subset of cytotrophoblast cells change their phenotype and invade deep into the uterine lining. These extravillous cytotrophoblast cells come into direct contact with the maternal decidual immune cells that include a small number of B lymphocytes, a moderate number of T lymphocytes and macrophages, and a voluminous number of natural killer cells. A subset of extravillous cytotrophoblast cells will invade directly into the maternal vasculature. These are the endovascular cytotrophoblast cells. They replace the endothelial cells of maternal vessels and transform the decidual vessels into the low-resistance, high-flow structures characteristic of a healthy, mature placenta.

Like the fetus, the placenta grows in size throughout pregnancy. At term, it is a large, beefy structure. Its maternal surface is covered with numerous cotyledons containing millions of villae. The fetal surface is covered with a smooth, glistening membrane called the amnion. The umbilical cord inserts almost perpendicularly into the fetal surface of the placenta.

Placental immunology

The maternal–fetal interface of the human hemochorial placenta allows direct exposure of fetally derived tissue to the maternal immune

Placental function

The placenta must supply the embryo and fetus with everything that it needs to grow and mature. Many complex systems exist within placental tissues to facilitate movement of nutrients into the fetus and wastes out. Driven by systemic blood pressure, maternal arterial blood spurts from the spiral arteries into the intervillous spaces and then disperses laterally (Fig. 17.2). The blood nearest the maternal decidua is under the least pressure and drains back into the maternal circulation. Only a fraction of the maternal blood vessels appears to spurt at any one time. This implies that that placental perfusion does not involve the entire placenta at any one time and that there is reserve capacity if a small separation from the uterine wall should occur.

At least four types of transport mechanisms move critical molecules from maternal blood, into the placenta and subsequently into the fetal circulation. Respiratory gas exchange occurs by **concurrent passive diffusion** down a concentration gradient as described by the Fick principle – its rate is proportional to the area of exchange, the diffusional permeability and the maternal and fetal blood flows. Although the oxygen content of umbilical cord blood coming directly from the placenta is low ($Po_2 = 28 - 32$ torr), the high affinity of fetal hemoglobin for oxygen assures that the fetal red blood cells are highly saturated with oxygen. Glucose, the primary metabolic fuel for the embryo and fetus, is transferred by **facilitated diffusion** involving classic GLUT transporters. Calcium enters the placenta through **active** cation **transport** whereas many amino acids are transported against concentration gradients coupled to sodium transport. Immunoglobulins of the immunoglobulin G (IgG) class enter the placenta through **endocytosis** following binding of the Fc end of the IgG molecules to membrane Fc receptors on trophoblasts.

18 The protein hormones of pregnancy

Figure 18.1 The protein hormones of pregnancy

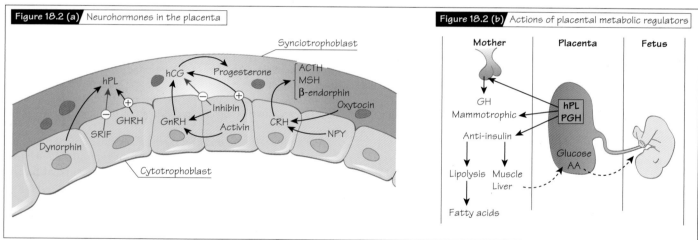

Figure 18.2 (a) Neurohormones in the placenta

Figure 18.2 (b) Actions of placental metabolic regulators

Placental production of protein hormones

The placenta is a very rich source of both protein and steroid hormones, only a few of which are unique to pregnancy (Fig. 18.1). These placental hormones are responsible for almost all the maternal and some of the fetal adaptations to pregnancy.

Human chorionic gonadotropin

Human chorionic gonadotropin (hCG) is a dimeric protein hormone whose structure is closely related to luteinizing hormone (LH) (Chapter 1). It is among the earliest products of the trophoblast cells of the embryo and is necessary to signal the maternal organism that conception has occurred. β-hCG mRNA can be detected in an eight-cell embryo, although intact hCG is not detectable in the maternal bloodstream or urine until 6 days after fertilization. hCG secretion is quantitatively related to the total mass of trophoblast in the placenta. Its concentration in the maternal serum approximately doubles every 2–3 days in early pregnancy; this can be used as a screen to differentiate

normal from abnormal pregnancies. Failure of the hCG concentrations to increase appropriately may indicate an abnormal implantation such as an ectopic (tubal) pregnancy or a nonviable intrauterine gestation. Higher than expected levels of hCG are seen with multiple gestations (Chapter 35) and molar pregnancies (Chapter 45).

The major biologic role of hCG is to "rescue" the corpus luteum of the ovary from its programmed demise 12–14 days after ovulation. Because of the close structural relationship of hCG to LH, hCG is able to bind to the LH receptor on luteal cells. hCG can therefore substitute for LH, supporting the corpus luteum when a pregnancy is present. Maintenance of the corpus luteum allows continued secretion of ovarian progesterone after day 14 postovulation and maintenance of the early pregnancy. Surgical removal of the corpus luteum without progesterone supplementation before the 9th menstrual week of pregnancy will result in a pregnancy loss. Administration of an antiprogestin such as RU-486 will have similar results. By 9 weeks' gestation (7 weeks after conception), the placenta has typically acquired sufficient cellular mass to supply the large amounts of progesterone necessary

The Reproductive System at a Glance, Fourth Edition. Linda J. Heffner and Danny J. Schust.

for pregnancy maintenance. Progesterone production is taken over by the placenta at this point and the corpus luteum could be removed without adverse effect on pregnancy maintenance. At the end of the first trimester, hCG also stimulates the fetal gonads to make the steroid hormones responsible for differentiation of the internal and external genitalia (Chapters 5 and 6).

Many of the hormones produced within the placenta result from a two-cell system that mimics the interactions between the neuroendocrine hypothalamus and the pituitary gland (Fig. 18.2a). For instance, gonadotropin-releasing hormone (GnRH) can be synthesized and secreted by the cytotrophoblast cells of the placenta. GnRH from the cytotrophoblast stimulates hCG production by the syncytiotrophoblast. As pregnancy progresses and the placenta becomes the major site of progesterone production, hCG's primary role changes from maintenance of the corpus luteum to maintenance of progesterone production by the syncytiotrophoblast. The serum level of hCG reflects this change by increasing to a maximum at about the 9th or 10th menstrual week of pregnancy and then decreasing to a much lower steady state level for the remainder of the pregnancy.

Human placental lactogen

Human placental lactogen (hPL) is a protein hormone produced exclusively by the placenta. It is structurally related to both prolactin and growth hormone (GH). When the peptide was originally isolated from the placenta, its biologic activity was assessed in animal models, where it has lactogenic activity. Although it was designated as a lactogen, lactogenic activity has not been clearly demonstrated in the human. Instead, hPL appears to function in metabolism (Fig. 18.2b). Its metabolic activities closely mimic those of GH, with which it shares 96% structural homology. Its effects on fat and carbohydrate metabolism include inhibition of peripheral glucose uptake, stimulation of insulin release by the pancreas and an increase in plasma free fatty acids. Prolonged fasting and hypoglycemia increase hPL production. During pregnancy, blood glucose decreases, insulin secretion increases and peripheral insulin resistance is enhanced. These metabolic changes are consistent with the presence of increased GH-like activity, possibly the effects of hPL. Another name for hPL is **human chorionic somatomammotropin (hCS)**.

In theory, the decreased maternal glucose utilization induced by hPL would ensure that a steady supply of glucose is available for fetal utilization. There is growing evidence that hPL is involved in regulating glucose homeostasis in the mother so that she can meet the nutritional demands of the fetus; however, successful pregnancies have been reported in the absence of hPL production by the placenta. In normal pregnancies, hPL production is directly proportional to placental mass and therefore rises steadily throughout pregnancy. At the end of gestation, over 1 g/day of hPL is produced by the placenta. This amount surpasses the production levels of any other protein hormone in either men or women.

Other hormones

Pituitary growth hormone of either maternal or fetal origin is not necessary for normal fetal growth. In fact, anencephalic fetuses lacking a pituitary gland and the offspring of women with GH deficiency will grow normally *in utero*. The placenta produces its own variant of GH protein, known as **placental growth hormone (PGH)**. PGH is a candidate hormone for regulating fetal growth. The placenta also produces somatotropin release inhibiting factor (SRIF), also known as somatostatin, that appears to affect HPL secretion by the placenta.

The cytotrophoblast cells and the syncytiotrophoblast secrete **corticotropin-releasing hormone (CRH)**, **neuropeptide Y (NPY)**, a CRH secretagogue, pro-opiomelanocortin (POM-C), the precursor to **adrenocorticotropic hormone (ACTH)** and **melanocyte stimulating hormone (MSH)**. Maternal CRH levels and placental CRH content rise in the last month of pregnancy. Glucocorticoids enhance CRH mRNA production by the placenta, suggesting a positive feedback system. It is hypothesized that placental CRH and ACTH may be involved in the timing of the onset of parturition. MSH appears to promote maturation of the fetal hypothalamic-pituitary-adrenal axis and has the secondary effect of darkening the maternal skin pigments. MSH induced darkening of the skin on the forehead, nose and cheeks of some pregnant women produces a mask-like appearance known as cholasma.

Maternal production of protein hormones

Placental hormones exert dramatic effects on the production and activities of nonplacental maternal protein hormones. For example, placental estrogen production stimulates the production of many hepatic proteins. Among these is thyroid-binding globulin (TBG). The increase in circulating TBG in the pregnant woman leaves less thyroid hormone free to circulate. Because free thyroid hormone exerts central negative feedback, this decrease in free thyroid hormone frees the hypothalamus to release thyroid-releasing hormone (TRH). Maternal pituitary thyroid-stimulating hormone (TSH) secretion increases in response to TRH and the maternal thyroid gland produces enough T_3 and T_4 to return the circulating levels to normal. Pregnant women therefore have higher levels of TBG, total T_3 and T_4, but normal amounts of free T_3 and T_4. This can cause confusion when interpreting thyroid function tests in pregnancy. It also means that pregnant women taking hormone replacement for thyroid gland deficiency often need to increase their dosage to maintain adequate free hormone levels.

Pituitary production of prolactin also increases dramatically as a result of estrogen stimulation in the pregnant woman. The number of lactotrophs in the pituitary gland doubles, thereby almost doubling the size and blood supply of the pituitary gland. This increase in size makes the pituitary gland particularly vulnerable to ischemic damage. Therefore, if postpartum hemorrhage and shock are not promptly treated, pituitary gland failure (Sheehan syndrome) may develop.

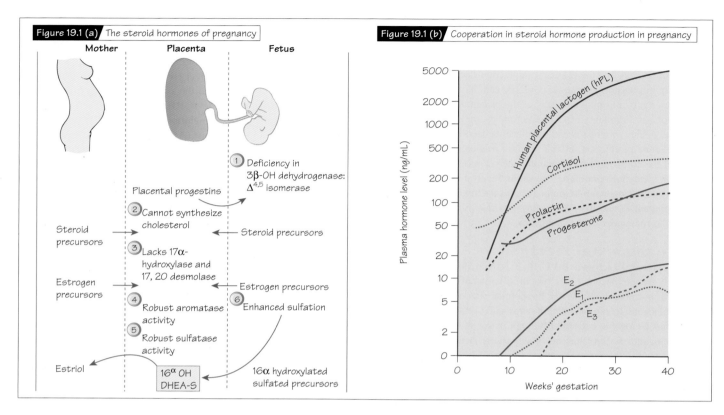

Figure 19.1 (a) The steroid hormones of pregnancy

Figure 19.1 (b) Cooperation in steroid hormone production in pregnancy

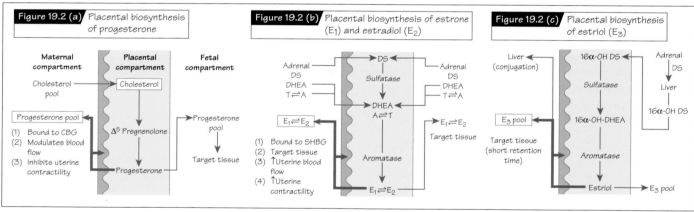

Figure 19.2 (a) Placental biosynthesis of progesterone

Figure 19.2 (b) Placental biosynthesis of estrone (E_1) and estradiol (E_2)

Figure 19.2 (c) Placental biosynthesis of estriol (E_3)

Steroid hormone production during pregnancy requires cooperation among maternal, fetal and placental organs and enzyme pathways (Fig. 19.1a). The fetus and the placenta each lack key steroidogenic enzymes and would be unable to synthesize certain steroid molecules if they existed in isolation. Interplay among fetus, placenta and the mother are essential to produce the full spectrum of steroidal products necessary for pregnancy maintenance. For example, the fetal adrenal gland has diminished 3β-hydroxysteroid dehydrogenase: Δ^{4-5} isomerase activity and therefore it secretes large amounts of the progesterone precursors, pregnenolone and dehydroepiandrosterone, and very little progesterone (Chapter 2). Because the fetus can synthesize so very little progesterone directly, it obtains its supplies from the placenta.

Because the syncytiotrophoblast layer of the placenta lacks a key enzyme, it cannot synthesize cholesterol from circulating acetate. To synthesize progesterone, the placenta requires cholesterol or pregnenolone from maternal or fetal sources. The vast majority arises from the maternal system and is transported to the placenta in the form of low density lipoprotein (LDL) cholesterol.

In contrast to the mother and placenta, the fetus has a remarkable ability to rapidly conjugate steroids with sulfates. Sulfation creates less potent steroids with more rapid clearance, characteristics that allow the fetus to be safely exposed to the high levels of circulating steroids seen during pregnancy. The fetal liver can efficiently hydroxylate steroid precursors and thereby provides the placenta with those

The Reproductive System at a Glance, Fourth Edition. Linda J. Heffner and Danny J. Schust.

hydroxylated steroids necessary for estrogen production. The placenta has almost no 17α-hydroxylase or 17,20 desmolase activity. For this reason, the precursors of the estrogens produced by the placenta must be supplied by the fetal or maternal systems. The placenta exhibits a robust ability to cleave sulfate groups from steroids. Placental sulfatase is integral to the formation of estrogens from fetal sulfated precursors. As the placenta lacks 17-α hydroxylase, all estriol produced during pregnancy arises from 17-α hydroxylated fetal precursors.

Progesterone

The corpus luteum of the ovary supplies progesterone until about 10 weeks' gestation. This supports pregnancy until placental progesterone production takes over in weeks 7–9 of gestation. The levels of 17α-hydroxyprogesterone produced by the corpus luteum rise in early pregnancy but fall by 10 weeks' gestation. After that time, placental production of progesterone dominates the maternal system and the placenta exhibits almost no 17α-hydroxylase activity.

Unlike other steroid-producing glands, the placenta lacks the enzymes to form cholesterol from acetate; therefore, progesterone produced by the syncytiotrophoblast is dependent on maternal cholesterol. hCG produced by the placenta supports the synthesis and secretion of progesterone within the placenta. Estrogens may also promote progesterone production by stimulating cholesterol uptake by the placenta and placental enzymatic conversion of cholesterol to pregnenolone. As a result, very large amounts of progesterone are produced and secreted by the placenta into the maternal bloodstream. This progesterone is active locally within the uterus, where it maintains the decidual lining of the uterus and relaxes the smooth muscle cells of the myometrium. It also has peripheral effects upon vascular smooth muscle and other organs that must adapt to the demands of pregnancy (Chapters 20 and 21).

Estrogens

The placenta can efficiently aromatize androgen precursors to estrogens because it expresses abundant amounts of the enzyme aromatase. All three of the major estrogens, estrone (E_1), estradiol (E_2) and estriol (E_3), are produced in the placenta; however, their androgen precursors arise from different sources (Fig. 19.2). Because placental aromatase is so abundant, it is not rate-limiting. Therefore, the relative amounts of each estrogen produced are determined by the amounts of substrate delivered to the placenta. The **major androgen precursor for placental estrogen production is dehydroepiandrosterone sulfate (DHEA-S)**. DHEA-S is an adrenal androgen and the majority supplied to the placenta originates in the maternal adrenal gland. In the placenta, DHEA-S is converted to DHEA by the abundant placental sulfate-cleaving enzyme, sulfatase. Maternal DHEA is then converted to androstenedione, then testosterone and finally to estrone and estradiol (Chapter 2). A very small amount of fetal DHEA-S is also utilized by the placenta to produce estrone and estradiol. **However, the majority of fetal DHEA-S is converted to estriol in the placenta**. To accomplish this, most of the fetal DHEA-S first undergoes 16-hydroxylation in the fetal liver. When the fetal 16α-OH-DHEA-S reaches the placenta, the placental sulfatase cleaves the sulfate side chain. 16α-OH DHEA is further metabolized and aromatized within the placenta to estriol. Estriol, which is not produced by the human ovary, is a relatively weak estrogen, but when produced at the high levels seen in pregnancy it can have dramatic estrogenic effects. The amount of estriol produced by the placenta far exceeds that of estrone and estradiol, making **placental estriol of fetal origin the major placental estrogen**.

Like progesterone, most of the estrogen produced by the placenta is found in the maternal compartment (uterus and bloodstream). Unlike its other estrogenic activities, estriol appears to be as effective as estradiol and estrone in increasing uteroplacental blood flow. Its relatively weak estrogenic effects on other organ systems make it highly effective in this single important pregnancy function. Its unique production from a fetal substrate also permits fetal regulation of uteroplacental blood flow. Uteroplacental blood flow is an important determinant of fetal growth and well-being.

Fetal adrenal physiology

By about 9 weeks' gestation, the fetal adrenal gland has developed an inner fetal zone and a very thin outer definitive zone. The latter will develop into the adrenal cortex in the adult. Approximately 80% of the gland is composed of the inner fetal zone. The fetal adrenal gland functions independently of adrenocorticotropic hormone (ACTH) until nearly 15–16 weeks' gestation. During this pre-ACTH phase, the fetal adrenal is thought to respond to hCG. After this time, it is controlled by ACTH secreted by the fetal pituitary gland. The fetal adrenal gland increases in size until about 24 weeks' gestation. It undergoes another impressive growth spurt at 34–35 weeks. 3β-hydroxysteroid dehydrogenase activity is limited in the fetal zone and therefore its major secretory products are DHEA and DHEA-S. These serve as the major substrates for circulating maternal estrogens. In fact, circulating maternal estrogen levels reflect the size of the fetal adrenal. Fetal ACTH control of its adrenals is assured by the presence of high levels of estrogen during pregnancy (Fig. 19.1b). Placental estrogens activate placental 11β-hydroxysteroid dehydrogenase. This in turn metabolizes maternal cortisol, allowing little to reach the fetal circulation.

Maternal adrenal function and salt metabolism

During pregnancy, the zona fasciculata of the maternal adrenal gland increases in size at the expense of the other adrenal cortical zones. In response, maternal glucocorticoid secretion increases, with significant elevations in maternal levels of circulating cortisol. Elevated estrogen levels also drive an increase in the production of cortisol-binding globulin. Still, an increase in the level of circulating free cortisol accompanies the increase in total cortisol. An increase in maternal plasma renin activity and angiotensinogen production results in an increase in plasma aldosterone levels during pregnancy. This results in elevated sodium retention and is partially responsible for the notable increase in maternal vascular volume.

Figure 20.1 Maternal physiologic adaptations to pregnancy

Maternal physiology must adapt in response to a series of demands attendant to pregnancy (Fig. 20.1). The pregnant woman needs to increase her circulating blood volume to supply nutrients to the fetus and to support amniotic fluid production. She must clear fetal waste products and protect her pregnancy from systemic perturbations, including starvation or medication ingestion. She must meet fetal and placental nutritional demands for glucose, amino acids and oxygen. The maternal system must adapt to allow for timely onset of labor and for protection of the mother from cardiovascular insults at the time of delivery. It must also prepare to support nourishment of the infant after delivery. All maternal organ systems are affected to some degree.

Cardiovascular system

During the first two trimesters of pregnancy, maternal circulating blood volume increases 40% (3500 cm^3 expands to 5000 cm^3) with the largest expansion occurring during the second trimester (Fig. 20.2). The functions of pregnancy-induced hypervolumia are to meet the demands of the enlarged uterus with its greatly hypertrophied vascular system, to provide nutrients to the growing placenta and fetus, to protect both mother and fetus from impaired venous return in certain postures, and to ensure that the mother does not suffer any adverse effects from the obligatory blood loss at delivery.

The increase in plasma volume results from a combination of a modest (10 mOsm/kg) decrease in plasma osmolality and from water retention through enhanced activity of the renin–angiotensin system. Placental estrogen increases hepatic production of angiotensinogen, and estrogen and progesterone together increase renal production of the proteolytic enzyme, renin. Renin cleaves angiotensinogen to form angiotensin I, which converts into angiotensin II (AII) in the lung and elsewhere. The increased amounts of AII act on the zona glomerulosa of the adrenal gland to increase aldosterone production. Aldosterone promotes volume expansion through sodium and water retention. Oxygen-carrying capacity must be maintained in the presence of this increase in circulating blood volume. Iron absorption increases to meet the demand for increased hemoglobin during volume expansion.

A loss of peripheral vascular responsiveness to AII accompanies the increase in circulating blood volume. AII is a potent vasoconstrictor and loss of AII responsivity results in a drop in maternal blood pressure during the early second trimester. This relative hypotension is seen in most pregnant women despite elevated AII levels. Maternal blood pressure slowly rises to prepregnancy levels by the third trimester. Progesterone promotes overall smooth muscle relaxation and is thereby partially responsible for alterations in maternal blood pressure. Production of prostacyclin, the principal endothelial prostaglandin, also increases during pregnancy and has been implicated in the development of angiotensin resistance.

Immediately following delivery of the fetus and placenta, a venous "autotransfusion" from the extremities, pelvis and empty uterus into the right heart occurs. Women with a normal cardiovascular system tolerate this event well but it is a major challenge for women with mitral valve stenosis and Eisenmenger syndrome in whom the increased venous return can result in pulmonary edema and hypoxia.

Respiratory system

An increase in tidal volume, minute ventilatory volume and minute O$_2$ uptake develops in pregnant women. These changes allow for increased oxygen delivery to the fetus and the periphery. They also cause a mild

The Reproductive System at a Glance, Fourth Edition. Linda J. Heffner and Danny J. Schust.

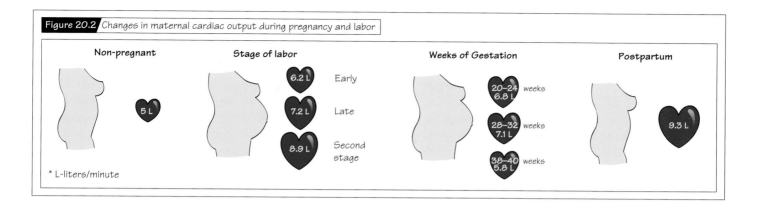

Figure 20.2 Changes in maternal cardiac output during pregnancy and labor

Non-pregnant

5 L

Stage of labor

6.2 L — Early

7.2 L — Late

8.9 L — Second stage

Weeks of Gestation

20–24 weeks 6.8 L

28–32 weeks 7.1 L

38–40 weeks 5.8 L

Postpartum

9.3 L

* L-liters/minute

maternal respiratory alkalosis that is compensated for by increased renal bicarbonate excretion. Progesterone may be responsible for many of these changes. The decrease in plasma bicarbonate shifts the O_2 dissociation curve to the left and increases the affinity of maternal hemoglobin for oxygen (the Bohr effect). This decreases the O_2 releasing capacity of the maternal blood which is offset by an increase in 2,3-diphosphoglycerate induced by the increase in pH. This shifts O_2 dissociation curve back to the right. Fetal hemoglobin binds O_2 at a lower partial pressure than maternal adult hemoglobin. The net result of these changes is to favor transfer of O_2 from mother to fetus within the placenta and to facilitate CO_2 (waste) transfer back from the fetus to the mother.

Many pregnant women have the sensation of shortness of breath in the absence of pathology. This physiologic dyspnea may be the result of decreased pCO_2. It is important to note that the blood gas pH of a pregnant woman should be in the alkalotic range with a decrease in pCO_2 and bicarbonate and, if not, requires further investigation.

Kidney and urinary tract

Maternal glomerular filtration rate (GFR) and renal plasma flow (RPF) begin to increase in early pregnancy. By midpregnancy, maternal GFR has increased by as much as 50%; it remains elevated throughout gestation. In contrast, maternal RPF begins to decrease in the third trimester. As a result, the renal filtration fraction increases during the last third of pregnancy. Because of the increased GFR, serum creatinine and urea are lower in pregnancy than in the nonpregnant state. Creatinine clearance is increased.

A 60–70% increase in the filtered load of sodium also accompanies the increased GFR. Progesterone appears to cause some sodium wastage by interfering with normal sodium resorption in the proximal renal tubule. In response, aldosterone increases proportionately to levels that are 2–3 times normal. Renal medullary prostaglandin E_2 synthesis also increases in late pregnancy, enhancing sodium natriuresis.

The relatively fixed renal tubular reabsorptive capacity, in combination with an increased GFR, causes a decrease in the reabsorption of glucose from the proximal tubule of the pregnant woman's kidney. Glucose is therefore detectable in the urine of about 15% of healthy pregnant women. Still, any pregnant woman exhibiting glycosuria should be evaluated for diabetes.

The volume of urine contained in the renal pelves and ureters can double in the latter half of pregnancy. The renal collecting system dilates during pregnancy as a result of mechanical obstruction by the pregnant uterus combined with the relaxing effects of progesterone upon smooth muscle. This dilatation decreases the speed of urine passage through the renal system and increases the maternal risk of developing acute kidney infections.

Hematologic system

Pregnant women are mildly anemic. Maternal hemoglobin production and total red blood cell mass increase during pregnancy in response to elevated erythropoietin production. Maternal vascular volume increases to a greater extent. The result is a mild maternal dilutional anemia that protects the mother from excess hemoglobin loss at delivery. The iron requirements of normal pregnancy must satisfy both maternal and fetal red cell production requirements and total about 1.0 g. Most is needed during the second half of pregnancy. Amounts of iron absorbed from diet alone, as well as any mobilized from maternal stores, may be insufficient to meet the demand.

Pregnant women develop a modest leukocytosis that can become quite marked during labor and postpartum. The etiology of the mild leukocytosis of early pregnancy is unclear. That seen during labor, however, resembles the leukocytosis associated with strenuous exercise, during which previously sequestered white cells re-enter the active circulation.

Pregnant women are hypercoagulable. Increased coagulability develops because of the increased procoagulant synthesis in the liver (Chapter 21). Up to 8% of women will develop a mild thrombocytopenia (<150 000 platelets/ml). This typically does not result in a bleeding diathesis. The mechanism by which the thrombocytopenia develops is unknown.

Skin

Circulating melanotrophic hormone (MSH) is increased during pregnancy as a result of the increased production of the precursor molecule pro-opiomelanocortin (POM-C) (Chapter 18). MSH causes darkening on the skin across the cheeks (chloasma or pregnancy mask) and darkening of the linea alba, the slightly pigmented line on the skin that runs from the navel to the pubis. Hair may also appear to fall out in clumps because of synchronization of hair follicle growth cycles during pregnancy.

㉑ Maternal adaptations to pregnancy: II

Thyroid gland

Maternal thyroid hormone is critical for normal embryonic and fetal development. Among the hepatic proteins stimulated by the elevated circulating levels of estrogen in pregnancy is thyroid-binding globulin (TBG). The increased TBG results in a decrease in circulating free T_3 and T_4 that will stimulate thyroid-stimulating hormone (TSH) production by the pituitary gland, thereby increasing the production of thyroxine by the thyroid gland. The alfa subunit of human chorionic gonadotropin (hCG) also appears to stimulate the thyroid gland, thereby assuring a timely increase in thyroxine production with pregnancy onset.

Interpretation of thyroid tests in pregnancy can be confusing because of the increased TBG. Total T_3 and T_4 will be elevated as will T_3 resin uptake (T_3RU), the indirect measure of total thyroxine binding capacity. Because of these changes, thyroid testing in pregnancy should rely on measurements of serum TSH and/or free T_3 and T_4.

Gastrointestinal tract

Pregnancy is a potentially diabetogenic state. It is a **state of relative hyperinsulinism with peripheral insulin resistance.** The high maternal levels of estrogen, progesterone and human placental lactogen (hPL) cause hypertrophy, hyperplasia and hypersecretion of insulin by the beta islet cells of the pancreas. Still, many pregnant women show prolonged hyperglycemia after meals. In addition, most pregnant women exhibit: (i) exaggerated insulin release in response to glucose infusion; (ii) reduced peripheral uptake of glucose; and (iii) suppressed glucagon secretion. Taken together, these traits characterize insulin resistance. The mechanism(s) for insulin resistance in pregnancy are not well understood. The growth hormone-like activity of hPL may be responsible. In addition, hPL may also promote lipolysis and liberation of free fatty acids that facilitate tissue resistance to insulin. These metabolic changes ensure a continuous supply of glucose for transfer to the fetus. Women at increased lifetime risk for developing type 2 diabetes mellitus (DM) will often develop a condition known as gestational diabetes mellitus (GDM). The presence of GDM confers a sevenfold risk of future type 2 DM. The same mechanisms that ensure a continuous supply of fetal glucose produce an "accelerated starvation" profile during fasting. Fasted pregnant women are relatively hypoglycemic and have higher circulating free fatty acids, triglycerides and cholesterol. Prolonged fasting or persistent vomiting in pregnant women can rapidly lead to ketonemia.

High maternal levels of circulating estrogens increase the synthesis of hepatic proteins. These include procoagulants, bile acids and multiple hormone binding proteins. The procoagulants most markedly elevated are factors I (fibrinogen), VII, VIII, IX and X. The higher circulating concentrations of clotting cascade proteins protect the mother from excessive blood loss at the time of delivery; however, they also predispose pregnant and postpartum women to venous thrombosis and embolism. Estrogens also stimulate the cytochrome P450 oxidative pathway in the liver. This increases the production of steroid precursors and can dramatically alter drug metabolism. The latter effect necessitates careful monitoring of the maternal plasma drug levels of many commonly used therapeutics. Most notable are the anticonvulsants and antibiotics.

The calcium requirements of the developing fetal and neonatal skeleton produce a profound maternal calcium stress during pregnancy and lactation. Maternal plasma parathyroid hormone (PTH) concentrations rise despite a minimal decrease in circulating free calcium. Intestinal absorption of calcium is enhanced by an increase in circulating 1,25-dihydroxyvitamin D_3, the active metabolite of vitamin D. 1,25-$(OH)_2$-D_3 increases for two reasons: (i) PTH increases the hepatic synthesis of 25-(OH)-D_3, and (ii) the activity of 1α-hydroxylase increases in pregnancy. In nonpregnant women and men, conversion of 25-(OH)-D_3 to the 1,25 active form is limited by the activity of 1α-hydroxylase, the final converting enzyme in D_3 metabolism. 1α-hydroxylase is typically present only in the kidney but, in pregnancy, it is produced by both the decidua and placenta. This ensures an adequate amount of active D_3 to optimize dietary calcium absorption during pregnancy. If dietary calcium intake is adequate, minimal mobilization of maternal bone calcium occurs. If it is not, fetal and neonatal skeletal mineralization will proceed at the expense of maternal bone density.

Progesterone relaxes smooth muscle and thereby affects all parts of the gastrointestinal tract during pregnancy. Gastric emptying is delayed, as is movement of digested material along the remainder of the tract. Gallbladder emptying is slower and bile tends to sludge in the bile duct and common duct. Minor disorders of the gastrointestinal tract are very common in pregnancy. These include nausea, vomiting, constipation and heartburn.

Nutritional requirements of pregnancy

The nutritional requirements of pregnancy are complex and include **water, oxygen, macronutrients (glucose, essential amino acids and fatty acids) and micronutrients (vitamins and minerals).** Water is necessary for volume support of the fetus and placenta and for the increase in maternal blood volume (Chapter 20), oxygen for efficient energy production as ATP, macronutrients for energy production and body growth, and micronutrients for regulating the expression of developmental genes and subsequent tissue functions.

Total maternal water retention at term is approximately 6.5 L with approximately 3.5 L in the fetus, placenta and amniotic fluid and another 3.0 L in the expanded uterus, breasts and blood volume (Table 21.1). Glucose is the predominant source of reduced nicotinamide adenine dinucleotide phosphate (NADPH), which is an essential cofactor for antioxidative enzymes and diverse metabolic pathways in all cell types. Fetal glucose is primarily derived from the uptake and transport of maternal glucose by the placenta. Amino acids serve as building blocks for proteins and as essential precursors of hormones, neurotransmitters, nitric oxide (NO), creatine, glutathione, carnitine and polyamines. Essential amino acids cannot be synthesized by either mother or fetus and must be derived from high quality protein foods or supplements. Long chain fatty acids readily cross the placenta from mother to fetus where they serve as major metabolic fuels.

The three most important dietary minerals in pregnancy are **calcium, iodine and iron.** Besides being a major component of the fetal skeleton, cytoskeleton and teeth, **calcium** is also required for calcium activated enzymes involved in digestion, cell–cell adhesion, blood clotting, intracellular proteolysis and NO synthesis. **Iodine** is required

The Reproductive System at a Glance, Fourth Edition. Linda J. Heffner and Danny J. Schust.

	Weight gained (kg)	Weight gained (lb)
Table 21.1 Average pregnancy weight gain in healthy populations		
Placenta	0.7	1.5
Fetus	3.2–3.6	7.0–8.0
Amniotic fluid	0.9	2.0
Uterine hypertrophy	0.9	2.0
Breast enlargement	0.45–1.4	1.0–3.0
Blood:		
Cellular components	1.4–1.8	3.0–4.0
Plasma	0.9–1.4	2.0–3.0
Fat stores	2.7–3.6	6.0–8.0
Total	11.15–14.3	24.5–31.5

for thyroid hormone synthesis; thyroid hormones, in turn, are required for normal fetal neuronal development. Iodine requirements in pregnancy increase by ~30%, -from 150 to 225 µg/day. Severe maternal iodine deficiency is associated with cretinism and milder forms of deficiency with impaired cognitive development of the infant. **Iron**, the most abundant trace element in the body, is a component of hemoglobin, myoglobin and cytochromes. Thus, physiologic levels of iron are necessary for (i) oxygen binding, transport, storage and sensing; (ii) metabolism of glucose, proteins and lipids; (iii) mitochondrial electron transport and ATP production; (iv) DNA synthesis; (v) immunity; and (vi) antioxidant activity. Iron requirements in pregnancy almost double from 15 to 27 mg/day.

Clinical observations and animal studies have demonstrated that **vitamins A, B6, B12, D and folate** have a major impact on pregnancy outcomes. Pyridoxal phosphate, the active form of vitamin B6, folic acid and vitamin B12 are of significance to fetal development because of their role in one-carbon-unit metabolism. **Folate** is essential to normal embryonic and fetal development and growth. Folate deficiency in early pregnancy can disrupt neural tube formation; supplementation has been shown in clinical studies to reduce the incidence of neural tube defects.

The absolute quantities of macro- and micronutrients required during pregnancy in a given woman will vary depending on her pre-pregnancy nutritional status. Anemic women will require more iron. It is estimated that only half of women in developed countries have adequate dietary intake of micronutrients; hence, prenatal supplements are typically recommended. In the underdeveloped and developing world, supplementation is even more critical but often absent. Women with a low body mass index (BMI) will require more calories during pregnancy to support normal fetal growth than women with a normal BMI. The interaction between prepregnancy nutritional status and caloric intake during pregnancy was first recognized when the offspring born during a 6-month famine in the Netherlands near the end of World War II were followed into adulthood. The offspring of previously well-nourished women who experience caloric deprivation during pregnancy are at increased risk of being born small for gestational age (SGA) and developing hypertension, coronary heart disease and type 2 DM in adulthood. If the woman is undernourished entering pregnancy, the growth restriction and subsequent abnormalities are more severe and earlier in onset. It is hypothesized that maternal undernutrition leads to development of a "**thrifty phenotype**" in the fetus that reallocates energy and nutrition to favor development of

organs critical to immediate survival. Obesity and metabolic and cardiovascular abnormalities subsequently develop when these individuals are raised in an environment with a great abundance of high energy foods. Overweight or obese women are at risk of delivering both SGA and excessively large infants who also have an increased risk of obesity in childhood and adulthood.

The biologic basis for these **fetal origins of adult disease** appears to be **epigenetic programming**, the stable and inheritable alterations of genes through covalent modifications of their DNA and core histones without changes in the DNA sequence. Recent studies indicate that abnormal fetal growth is associated with hypomethylation or hypermethylation of genes involved with the synthesis and regulation of the insulin-like growth factor (IGF) system. Changes in leptin secretion and sensitivity that affect eating may also be involved.

Immune system

The immunology of pregnancy is fairly complicated and may vary fairly significantly over the course of gestation. The processes of implantation and parturition are inflammatory in nature, yet maternal immune reactivity over the majority of pregnancy requires a significant level of immune tolerance. The fetus represents a hemi-allograft in a typically immunocompetent host, however, graft rejection usually does not occur. Although the fetus is recognized by the maternal immune system, the incited allo-response is not cytotoxic in healthy pregnancies. Rather, there is an increase in maternal regulatory T helper cell (T reg) number and activity that promotes tolerance to the recognized fetus-specific antigen. Further, normally cytotoxic CD8+ T cells at the maternal-fetal interface tend to be deficient in the expression of cytolytic molecules such as perforin and granzyme B.

Several additional factors are known to be involved in maternal immune tolerance to the developing fetus; many remain to be discovered. For example, the fetally-derived placenta does not express classic transplantation antigens that would typically provoke rejection. This includes major histocompatibility complex (MHC) class II and most MHC class I products. Tolerogenic changes in maternal immunity do not come without costs. For example, pregnant women experience a higher attack rate and more severe or prolonged disease upon exposure to certain viral pathogens (e.g. varicella/chickenpox).

Maternal antibody-mediated immunity is actively transferred to the fetus beginning at approximately 16 weeks' gestational age when receptors for the Fc region of immunoglobulin G (IgG) appear in the placenta.

Labor

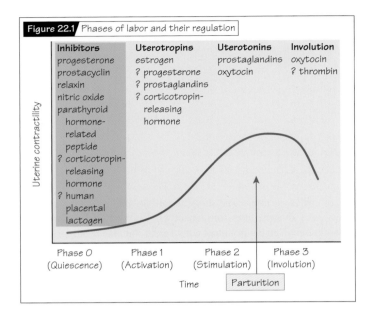

Figure 22.1 Phases of labor and their regulation

Inhibitors	Uterotropins	Uterotonins	Involution
progesterone	estrogen	prostaglandins	oxytocin
prostacyclin	? progesterone	oxytocin	? thrombin
relaxin	? prostaglandins		
nitric oxide	? corticotropin-		
parathyroid	releasing		
hormone-	hormone		
related			
peptide			
? corticotropin-			
releasing			
hormone			
? human			
placental			
lactogen			

Uterine contractility

Phase 0 (Quiescence) Phase 1 (Activation) Phase 2 (Stimulation) Phase 3 (Involution)

Time   Parturition

Labor is the process by which the fetus and its supporting placenta and membranes pass from the uterus to the outside world. **It is defined as regular uterine contractions that result in thinning and dilatation of the cervix so that the products of conception can pass out of the uterus.** Labor involves three key processes: (i) a switch in myometrial activity, from a longer lasting, low-frequency irregular contraction pattern called "contractures" to the frequent, high-intensity, regular pattern known as "contractions"; (ii) softening and dilatation of the cervix; and (iii) rupture of the fetal membranes. Although labor may first become apparent with the isolated appearance of any of these three elements, the physiologic events that produce them typically occur simultaneously.

Phases of labor

It is useful to consider labor as a series of four physiologic phases, characterized by the release of the myometrium from the inhibitory effects of pregnancy and the activation of stimulants of myometrial contractility (Fig. 22.1). Phase 0 comprises the majority of pregnancy. During this phase, the uterus is maintained in a state of quiescence by one or more inhibitors of contractility. Candidate inhibitors include progesterone, prostacyclin, nitric oxide, parathyroid hormone-related peptide (PTHrP), calcitonin gene-related peptide, relaxin, adrenomedullin and vasoactive intestinal peptide (VIP). Near the end of a normal pregnancy, the uterus undergoes the process of activation (Phase 1). During activation, a number of contraction-associated proteins increase under the influence of estrogen. These proteins include myometrial receptors for prostaglandins and oxytocin, membranous ion channels and connexin-43, a key component of gap junctions. The increase in myometrial gap junctions during activation will electrically couple adjacent myometrial cells and maximize the coordination of contraction waves that move from the uterine fundus to the cervix. Phase 2 of labor is called stimulation. During stimulation, oxytocin and stimulatory prostaglandins (PGs) such as PGE$_2$ and PGF$_{2\alpha}$ can

induce contractions in the previously primed uterus. The cervix dilates. The fetus, membranes and placenta are expelled from the uterus in a process called parturition. Phase 3 of labor follows parturition and is called involution. During involution, sustained contraction of the uterus promotes necessary hemostasis and eventually reduces the massively enlarged postpartum uterus to a size only slightly larger than its prepregnant state.

Initiation of labor

The average human gestation lasts 280 days (40 weeks) from the beginning of the last menstrual period. Exactly what triggers human labor is unknown. Still, like other species that bear live young, the fetoplacental unit appears to control at what point in gestation labor will occur while maternal signals determine the time of day that it will start. The mechanisms used by the fetoplacental unit to initiate labor vary from species to species. Humans mimic the mechanisms used by other primates much more closely than those used by more distantly related mammals.

Sheep and rodents rely on progesterone withdrawal for labor initiation. In stark contrast, the initiation of labor in primates involves increases in placental estrogen synthesis (Fig. 22.2). Seemingly, this estrogen must be produced by the placenta, because systemic infusion of estrogen does not induce labor at term. Rather, infused androstenedione will induce contractions and this effect can be blocked by inhibiting aromatase activity. Placental aromatase activity (Chapters 2 and 19) increases at term. This is accompanied by an increase in production of adrenal androgen precursors (e.g., androstenedione) by the fetus. Both support increased placental estrogen production.

The stimulus for the increase in fetal adrenal androgen production near term is not known. It does not appear to arise from the fetal hypothalamus (corticotropin-releasing factor, CRH) or fetal pituitary adrenocorticotropic hormone (ACTH) because absence of appropriate brain formation in anencephalic fetuses does not prolong pregnancy. Rather, the stimulus is likely to be placental. Placental CRH is an excellent candidate. Placental CRH is biochemically identical to maternal and fetal hypothalamic CRH but differs in its regulation. Glucocorticoids exert negative feedback on the synthesis and release of hypothalamic CRH, but stimulate placental CRH. Placental CRH appears to stimulate fetal ACTH production and fetal adrenal steroid synthesis (e.g., androstenedione production). It may also have local effects within the uterus, fostering placental vasodilatation, prostaglandin production and myometrial contractility.

In all species, an increase in prostaglandin synthesis by the decidua and the fetal membranes constitutes the final common pathway in labor. Human uterine tissues are selectively enriched with arachidonic acid, an essential fatty acid that is the obligate precursor of those prostaglandins most important in labor: PGE and PGF$_{2\alpha}$. Both cyclooxygenase enzymes, COX-1 and COX-2, are expressed in the uterus. COX-2, the inducible form of the enzyme, appears to be sensitive to glucocorticoid induction. Evidence for the role of prostaglandins in labor includes observations that: (i) the concentrations of PGs in amniotic fluid, maternal plasma and maternal urine are increased before the onset of labor; (ii) administration of PGs at any stage of pregnancy can initiate labor; (iii) PGs can induce cervical ripening and

The Reproductive System at a Glance, Fourth Edition. Linda J. Heffner and Danny J. Schust.

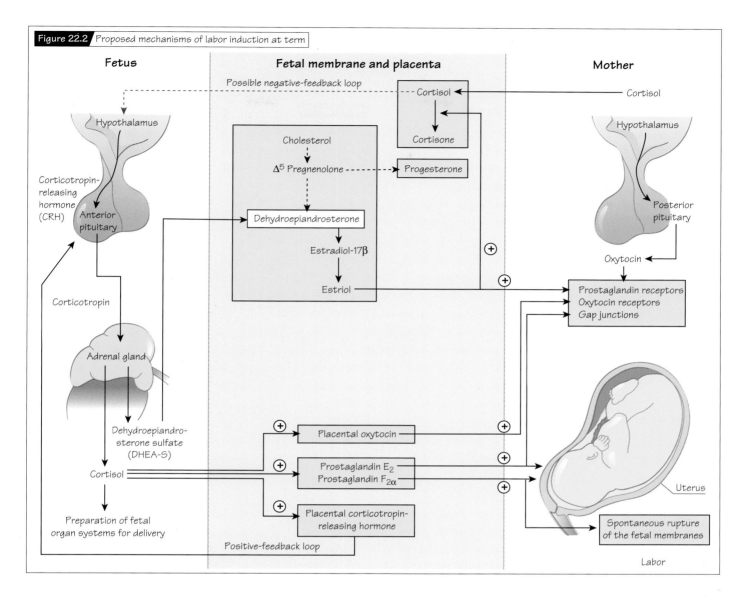

Figure 22.2 Proposed mechanisms of labor induction at term

Fetus | Fetal membrane and placenta | Mother

Possible negative-feedback loop

Hypothalamus

Corticotropin-releasing hormone (CRH)

Anterior pituitary

Corticotropin

Adrenal gland

Dehydroepiandro-sterone sulfate (DHEA-S)

Cortisol

Preparation of fetal organ systems for delivery

Cholesterol

Δ^5 Pregnenolone

Dehydroepiandrosterone

Estradiol-17β

Estriol

Cortisol

Cortisone

Progesterone

(+) Placental oxytocin

(+) Prostaglandin E$_2$
Prostaglandin F$_{2\alpha}$

(+) Placental corticotropin-releasing hormone

Positive-feedback loop

Cortisol

Hypothalamus

Posterior pituitary

Oxytocin

(+) (+) Prostaglandin receptors
Oxytocin receptors
Gap junctions

(+)
(+)

Uterus

Spontaneous rupture of the fetal membranes

Labor

---

uterine contractions; (iv) PGs increase myometrial sensitivity to oxytocin; and (v) inhibitors of PG synthesis can suppress contractions and prolong pregnancy (e.g., the COX inhibitor, indomethacin).

Like other smooth muscle cells, myometrial cells are triggered to contract by a rise in intracellular calcium (Ca^{2+}). Prostaglandins raise intracellular Ca^{2+} by increasing Ca^{2+} influx across the cell membranes, by stimulating calcium release from intracellular stores and by enhancing myometrial gap junction formation.

Oxytocin, a posterior pituitary hormone, has an important role in labor. Oxytocin acts through its membrane receptor on myometrial cells to activate members of the G protein subfamily. These, in turn, activate phospholipase C and inositol triphosphate, causing a release of intracellular Ca^{2+}. Oxytocin seems to have a role in the maternal control of the time of day that labor will start. Several days to weeks before the onset of recognizable labor, myometrial activity switches away from contractures to contractions. This switch invariably occurs when the lights go off in the animal's environment and ensures that delivery will occur

when the mother is safely at rest away from predators. Nocturnally active animals will thus deliver during the day and vice versa. This circadian rhythm of uterine activity is accompanied by an increase in circulating oxytocin and in myometrial oxytocin receptors.

Oxytocin also has an important role in promoting expulsion of the fetus from the uterus after the cervix is fully dilated. In fact, the oxytocin concentrations in the maternal circulation do not begin to rise until the expulsive stage of labor begins. Still, the gradual increase in the concentrations of oxytocin receptor in the myometrium during the second half of pregnancy may allow for lower concentrations of oxytocin to effect myometrial contractions prior to the onset of expulsion. Oxytocin can induce prostaglandin production and gap junction formation within the uterus, suggesting that it may act in synergy with other factors to initiate labor. To this point, oxytocin can be used clinically to induce and to stimulate labor. The fetus, placenta and fetal membranes all make oxytocin that is selectively secreted toward the maternal compartment.

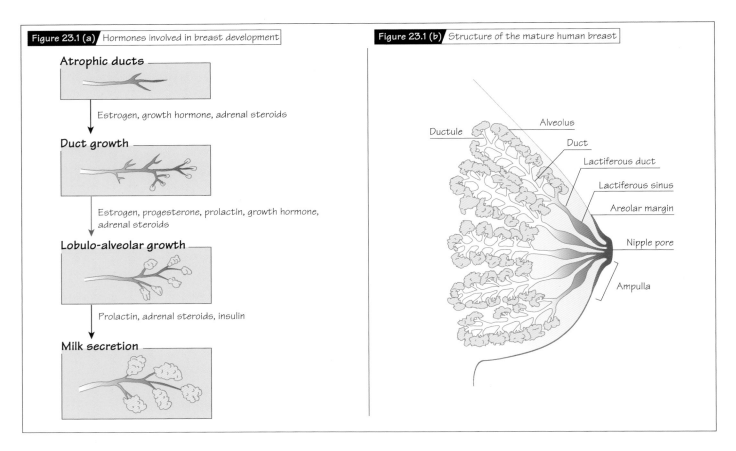

Figure 23.1 (a) Hormones involved in breast development

Atrophic ducts

Estrogen, growth hormone, adrenal steroids

Duct growth

Estrogen, progesterone, prolactin, growth hormone, adrenal steroids

Lobulo-alveolar growth

Prolactin, adrenal steroids, insulin

Milk secretion

Figure 23.1 (b) Structure of the mature human breast

Ductule
Alveolus
Duct
Lactiferous duct
Lactiferous sinus
Areolar margin
Nipple pore
Ampulla

Development of the breast

The human mammary gland is derived from ectoderm. It is first visible in the 4-week embryo as a bud or nodule of epithelial tissue appearing along a line known as the milk crest. In the more developed embryo, this crest extends from the midaxilla to the inguinal region and may be the site of supernumerary breasts or nipples in the adult. The rudimentary epithelial nodule first becomes buried in embryonic mesenchyme, where it undergoes further differentiation, apparently under the influence of paracrine signals from the mesenchyme. Secondary epithelial buds form cellular cords that elongate, bifurcate and cavitate. These cords become the excretory and lactiferous ducts of the mammary gland.

The human mammary gland is a compound tuboalveolar structure composed of 15–25 irregular lobes radiating out from the nipple (Fig. 23.1). Individual lobes are embedded in adipose tissue and separated by dense layers of connective tissue. Each lobe is further subdivided into lobules, connected to the nipple by lactiferous ducts. The lactiferous ducts are lined by a stratified squamous epithelium. Loose connective tissue (stroma) surrounds the lactiferous ducts and permits their ready distension during lactation.

At birth, the breast is rudimentary and consists almost entirely of primitive lactiferous ducts. Although it may secrete a few drops of milk, called "witch's milk," this secretory function is short-lived and the breast quickly becomes quiescent until puberty. At puberty, ovarian estrogens stimulate the lactiferous duct system to grow. After menarche,

exposure to cyclic progesterone induces further ductal growth and development of rudimentary lobules at the ends of the ducts. The breasts continue to grow for several years after menarche as the lactiferous ducts progressively subdivide, elongate and hollow out, and adipose tissue accumulates. However, complete lobular development and maturation will not occur in the absence of pregnancy.

At the beginning of pregnancy there is rapid growth and branching of the terminal portions of the rudimentary lobules under the influence of chorionic gondotropin. Vascularity increases dramatically. The pregnant woman often perceives these two changes as a "tingling" or "tension" in her breasts. This sensation begins shortly after conception and may last throughout the first trimester. At about 8 menstrual weeks of pregnancy, sustained progesterone exposures initiates complete alveolar differentiation. True glandular acini appear as hollow alveoli lined with a single layer of myoepithelial cells. The highly branched myoepithelial cells form a loose network surrounding the alveoli. The alveoli connect to the larger lactiferous ducts through intralobular ducts. Alveolar secretion begins in the second trimester of pregnancy. By the third trimester, an immunoglobulin-rich secretion is seen distending the alveoli.

While the role of ovarian steroids in breast development is clearly clinically established (prepubertal gonadal failure is associated with absence of breast development), animal models suggest that other hormones may also be involved in human breast development. Insulin exposure causes multiplication of epithelial cells and formation of

The Reproductive System at a Glance, Fourth Edition. Linda J. Heffner and Danny J. Schust.

lobuloalveolar architecture. Complete cytologic and functional differentiation of the epithelial cells lining the alveoli requires exposure to cortisol, insulin and prolactin. Receptors for growth factors such as insulin-like growth factor 1 (IGF-1) and epidermal growth factor (EGF) have been demonstrated on human mammary cells, suggesting an important role for their ligands in breast development and function.

Milk formation

Milk has more than 100 constituents. It is basically an emulsion of fat in a liquid phase that is isotonic with plasma. Mature human milk contains 3–5% fat, 1% protein, 7% lactose and 0.2% minerals, and delivers 60–75 kcal/dL. The principal class of human milk lipids is triglycerides. The main proteins in human milk are casein, α-lactalbumin, lactoferrin, immunoglobulin A, lysozyme and albumin. Casein and α-lactalbumin are specific milk proteins; α-lactalbumin is part of the enzyme complex lactose synthetase. Lactose is the primary sugar in human milk. Free amino acids, urea, creatinine and creatine are also present. Minerals include sodium, potassium, calcium, magnesium, phosphorus and chloride. As the composition of human breast milk continues to be studied, several peptide hormones, including EGF, transforming growth factor α (TGF-α), somatostatin and IGF-1 and IGF-2 have also been identified. The first milk secreted after delivery is called colostrum. It contains a higher protein content (largely immunoglobulins) and lower sugar content than subsequent secretions.

The alveolar epithelial cells that make milk are polarized, highly differentiated cells whose function is to accumulate, synthesize, package and export the components of milk. **At least four transcellular pathways** are required for appropriate **milk formation** within the alveolus of the breast. The first involves **secretion of monovalent cations and water**. Water is drawn across the alveolar cell by a concentration gradient generated by specific milk sugars; ions follow an electrochemical gradient. The second involves **receptor-mediated transport of immunoglobulins**. Immunoglobulin A (IgA) enters the epithelial cell after binding to its receptor, becomes internalized and is transported either to the Golgi apparatus or the apical membrane of the cell for secretion. The third pathway involves the **synthesis and transport of milk lipids**, which are synthesized in the cytoplasm and smooth endoplasmic reticulum. They then aggregate into droplets that coalesce to form larger fat globules. These are discharged from the apical part of the cell into the alveolar lumen. The final pathway involves **exocytosis of secretory vesicles containing specific milk proteins, calcium, phosphate, citrate and lactose**. These vesicles form in the Golgi apparatus. Here, casein, the specific milk protein, forms micelles with calcium and phosphate. The Golgi is impermeable to lactose. Because lactose is an osmotically active sugar, water is drawn into the Golgi and lactose content thereby determines the milk's liquid volume. A fifth pathway is required for milk formation: it is not transcellular, but paracellular. Immunoglobulins, such as IgA, plasma proteins and leukocytes can move between alveolar cells that have lost their tight junctions.

Regulation of milk production

Regulation of the quantity and content of breast milk is largely under hormonal control, with **prolactin** being the most important regulatory hormone in humans, although its actions require synergism with several others. Prolactin concentrations in the plasma rise steadily throughout pregnancy, from less than 20 ng/mL to over 200 ng/mL at term (Chapter 18). In breastfeeding women, basal serum prolactin levels remain elevated for about 4–6 weeks postpartum, then fall to nonpregnant levels despite continued lactation. For about the next 2 months, suckling causes spikes of prolactin release. Even with production of a litre or more of breast milk per day, this reflex is also gradually lost.

The pivotal role of prolactin in the initiation of breastfeeding was established by blocking secretion of the hormone from the pituitary using the dopamine agonist, bromocriptine. When bromocriptine is given to women shortly after delivery, prolactin levels drop precipitously to nonpregnant levels. Breast engorgement and lactation never occur. Estrogens can also be used to suppress lactation immediately postpartum, but they work through a different mechanism. After estrogen administration, prolactin levels remain quite elevated, but no milk is formed. Thus, estrogens inhibit the action of prolactin on the breast, which is probably why lactation does not occur before delivery. With delivery of the placenta, the source of the large amount of circulating estrogen is removed. Circulating estrogens drop precipitously and breast milk begins to form within 24–48 h. Bromocriptine administered later in the postpartum period also inhibits lactation, but only until the process no longer depends on prolactin.

Prolactin has several actions at the cellular level. It stimulates the synthesis of α-lactoglobulin and casein in breast tissue primed by insulin and cortisol. It stabilizes casein mRNA, prolonging its half-life eightfold. Prolactin stimulates milk fat synthesis and may be involved in sodium transport in mammary tissue. Interestingly, and unlike other polypeptide hormones, prolactin binding to its receptor does not stimulate adenylate cyclase activity.

The lactation reflex

Although prolactin is responsible for initiating milk production, milk delivery to the infant and lactation maintenance depend on mechanical stimulation of the nipple. The suckling stimulus is known as **milk ejection** or **letdown**. Although suckling is the major stimulus for milk letdown, the reflex can be conditioned. The cry or sight of an infant and preparation of the breast for nursing may cause letdown, while pain, embarrassment and alcohol can inhibit it.

The suckling reflex is initiated when sensory impulses originating in the nipple enter the spinal cord through its dorsal roots. A multisynaptic neural pathway ascends to the magnocellular supraoptic and paraventricular nuclei of the hypothalamus via activin-containing neurons in the nucleus solitarius tract. Impulse recognition results in episodic **oxytocin** release from the posterior pituitary. Oxytocin then stimulates the myoepithelial cells lining the milk ducts to contract, thereby causing milk "ejection."

A large surge in prolactin release is temporally associated with the episodic oxytocin release induced by nursing, but this surge will occur independently of the oxytocin changes. This transient pulse of prolactin induces milk formation for the next feeding. Smoking can inhibit this prolactin surge and cause a decrease in milk production.

The suckling reflex also affects the activity of the gonadotropin-releasing hormone (GnRH) pulse generator. Suckling inhibits gonadotropin release and ovulation does not typically occur. The effectiveness of lactation in suppressing gonadal function is directly related to the frequency and duration of nursing. Among the !Kung hunter-gatherers in Africa, the average interval between births is 44 months in spite of early postpartum resumption of coitus and lack of contraception. Mothers nurse about every 15 minutes and children are in immediate proximity to their mothers all day and night for 2 years or more.

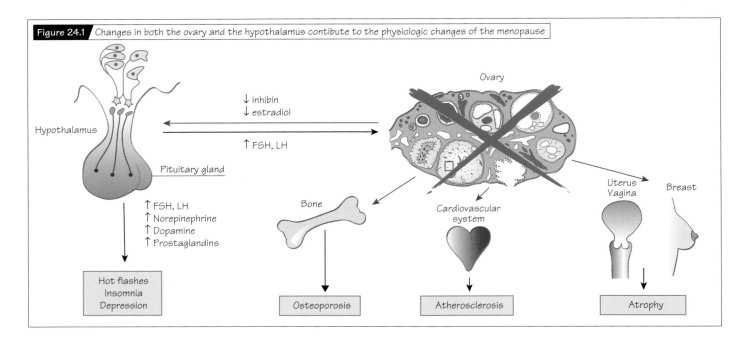

Figure 24.1 Changes in both the ovary and the hypothalamus contibute to the physiologic changes of the menopause

Menopause is a normal stage of life. Its health consequences have only become apparent as life expectancy has increased well beyond the 6th decade of life for women. It is estimated that women living in developed countries will live at least one-third of their lives after menopause. Functionally, menopause may be considered an "**estrogen withdrawal syndrome.**" It is recognizable by the loss of menses and, for most women, by the appearance of signs and symptoms such as hot flashes, insomnia, vaginal atrophy, decreased breast size and reduced skin elasticity. Osteoporosis and cardiovascular disease represent longer term consequences of estrogen deficiency (Fig. 24.1). Both are more indolent and less predictable than the early signs and symptoms of menopause.

Physiology of menopause

The postmenopausal ovary is small and essentially devoid of follicles. The appearance of the postmenopausal ovary, coupled with the observation that oophorectomy is associated with menopausal symptoms, led to the original theory that follicular depletion was responsible for menopause. More recent evidence suggests that menopause has origins in both the central nervous system and the ovary. In addition, men appear to experience a similar, albeit later and more subtle change, called andropause. Both changes can be referred to as "gonadopause" and associated mechanisms in the central nervous system and gonads seem to be quite extensive and to reflect the general aging process.

Fertility decreases dramatically in women beginning at about age 35 but accelerating after the age of 40. The accelerated fall after 40 may be the first sign of impending ovarian failure. Although ovarian follicles remain visible on ultrasound, attempts at artificial induction of ovulation with injected gonadotropins are largely unsuccessful after

about age 45 years. This suggests that a physiologic defect develops within the oocytes or follicles prior to their depletion. About 3–4 years before menopause is apparent, serum follicle-stimulating hormone (FSH) levels begin to rise subtly and ovarian estrogen, anti-Müllerian hormone, inhibin and progesterone production falls. Menstrual cycle length tends to decrease as the follicular phase progressively shortens. Ultimately, ovulation and menstruation cease entirely. The age of onset of menopause has changed very little over time – even the Ancient Greeks mention the age of 50 as typical. Age of menopause is affected by multiple factors. Maternal menopausal age is predictive of a daughter's menopausal age. Age of menarche does not affect age of menopause. Most agree that race and parity have no effect. Smokers enter menopause at an earlier age than nonsmokers.

Although ovarian failure is a major component of menopause, functional alterations also occur at the level of the pituitary. Changes arise in the intrinsic rhythms that control sleep and the neuroendocrine axes. Such changes in the circadian oscillator lead to diminished nocturnal melatonin secretion and altered sleep, decreased responsiveness of the gonadotropin axis to steroid feedback and decreased adrenal steroid production. Aging is also associated with a more general decline in central dopaminergic and noradrenergic neuronal function. Estrogen deficiency further exacerbates the dopamine deficiency by increasing the ratio of norepinephrine to dopamine.

During menopause, the decrease in ovarian estrogen and inhibin production reduces negative feedback signals to the pituitary and hypothalamus and results in a progressive rise in gonadotropin levels. Because inhibin acts exclusively to regulate FSH (Chapter 1), FSH levels rise disproportionately to luteinizing hormone (LH) levels. **When in doubt, persistent elevation of serum FSH levels confirms**

The Reproductive System at a Glance, Fourth Edition. Linda J. Heffner and Danny J. Schust.

56 © 2014 John Wiley & Sons, Ltd. Published 2014 by John Wiley & Sons, Ltd. Companion Website: www.ataglanceseries.com/reproduction

the diagnosis of menopause. Although ovarian estrogen production essentially ceases, the ovary continues to make the androgens testosterone and androstenedione. Most of this steroid biosynthesis occurs in the hilar cells of the medulla of the gland and very little occurs in the stroma. Hilar cells share a common embryologic origin with testicular Leydig cells, the main androgen-secreting cells in the male (Chapter 5).

Although ovarian estrogen production ceases at menopause, postmenopausal women are not completely estrogen deficient. Peripheral tissues such as fat, liver and kidney express the enzyme aromatase and can convert circulating androgens to estrogens. The major difference between direct ovarian estrogen secretion and peripheral conversion is that most of the estrogen produced by the latter process is estrone. Estrone is the estrogen produced from aromatization of androstenedione, the major androgen secreted by the postmenopausal ovary and adrenal gland (Chapter 2). Estrone is a very weak estrogen compared with estradiol. In the typical concentrations found in postmenopausal women, estrone does not provide protection against the long-term consequences of estrogen deficiency. Obese postmenopausal women are somewhat protected from this. Fat is a particularly rich source of aromatase activity and obese postmenopausal women can produce substantial amounts of estrone. These high quantities of endogenous estrone provide some protection against the risk of menopausal vasomotor symptoms and osteoporosis but at a cost. Prolonged exposure of the endometrium to estrogen stimulation that is unopposed by postovulatory progesterone will increase the risk for the development of endometrial hyperplasia and carcinoma (Chapter 42). The endometrium is never converted from proliferative physiology to secretory morphology and this unregulated growth favors neoplastic change. A similar risk of endometrial stimulation is present in women receiving estrogen alone for postmenopausal hormone replacement. For this reason, women who still have their uterus but require or choose postmenopausal estrogen replacement should also be given progesterone in a continuous or cyclic fashion.

Signs and symptoms
Hot flashes
Hot flashes or flushes occur in about 75% of menopausal women. Nocturnal hot flashes often wake a woman from sleep and may produce significant sleep deprivation or insomnia. During a hot flash most women note a sensation of pressure in their head followed by a flush of heat or burning. This sensation begins on the head or neck area and passes over the entire body. Sweating invariably accompanies the flush. While there are profound physiologic changes associated with hot flashes, the mechanism by which estrogen deficiency produces this symptom is not known. The physiologic changes include an initial increase in skin conductance and then temperature, a reflection of peripheral vasodilatation. Core body temperature subsequently drops by an average of 0.2°C. Circulating estrogen levels do not change before or after the flash but LH, cortisol, dehydroepiandrosterone (DHEA), androstenedione and the pro-opiomelanocortin (POM-C) derived peptides all do. It is believed that the hot flash represents an initial change in central thermoregulation that elicits a number of compensatory mechanisms. These mechanisms transiently raise, but ultimately reduce the core body temperature to the new set point. Central nervous system catecholamines are involved in hypothalamic temperature regulation and the impact of estrogen deficiency on noradrenergic neuronal function likely has a role in hot flashes. Some hypothesize that estrogen deficiency predisposes to vasodilatation within the hypothalamus. This results in an increase in hypothalamic

temperature and a response favoring a reduction in the core body temperature.

In addition to hot flashes, most menopausal women experience **vaginal atrophy and changes in their breasts and skin**. Vaginal atrophy can lead to decreased vaginal lubrication. This may be physically uncomfortable, may predispose to urinary tract infections and may result in dyspareunia during intercourse. These changes are directly related to the loss of estrogen stimulation in target tissues and can largely be reversed by estrogen replacement.

Bone changes
Bone loss in women actually begins at about age 30. It accelerates at menopause. The most rapid bone loss occurs in the first 3–4 years after menopause. Bone loss occurs more quickly in women who smoke and in very thin women. African-American race and fluoride treatment of the water supply are associated with a lower incidence of osteoporosis. The most common site of osteoporosis-related fractures is the vertebral body, an effect that may be noted clinically as back pain and the development of a "dowager's hump." The upper femur, humerus, ribs and distal forearm are also frequently affected by postmenopausal bone loss. Upper femoral fractures that involve the hip joint may be life-threatening because of an accompanying risk of venous thromboembolic disease.

Osteoporosis resulting from prolonged estrogen deficiency involves a reduction in the quantity of bone without alterations in its chemical composition. Bone formation by osteoblasts is normal in estrogen-deficient women but the rate of bone resorption by osteoclasts is increased. Trabecular bone is affected first, followed by cortical bone. Estrogen appears to antagonize the effects of parathyroid hormone (PTH) on calcium mobilization. This may occur as a direct effect of estrogen on bone because estrogen receptors have been found on bone cells in culture.

Cardiovascular changes
Estrogen receptors are present on blood vessels and estrogen appears to clinically decrease vascular resistance and increase blood flow. One potential mechanism by which estrogen may improve blood flow is through its demonstrated ability to decrease the production of endothelin, a potent vasoconstrictor, by vascular endothelium. Estrogen therapy is also associated with an increase in high-density lipoproteins and decrease in low-density lipoproteins. Despite these mechanistic findings, the results of several recent large population studies have suggested that postmenopausal hormone replacement therapy (HRT) may have untoward cardiovascular effects. These results need to be taken in context with risks and benefits weighed for a particular patient. For instance, one arm of the Women's Health Initiative, which is the largest randomized trial of HRT, showed that use of combinations of estrogen and progestin in the treatment of postmenopausal women resulted in seven additional cases of heart disease, eight pulmonary emboli, eight strokes and eight additional cases of breast cancer among 10 000 women treated for 1 year. At the same time, there were six fewer cases of colon cancer and five fewer hip fractures. This resulted in 20 women who were harmed by therapy out of 10 000 undergoing treatment. Although recent data have relaxed prohibitions somewhat, postmenopausal estrogen replacement regimens in the years after release of the results of the Women's Health Initiative have been severely retstricted, with most practitioners limiting therapy to the treatment of hot flashes and vaginal atrophy. When given, estrogen has typically been provided in the lowest dose and for the shortest duration possible. Alternative medications and delivery systems for postmenopausal hormone replacement are under investigation.

㉕ Contraception

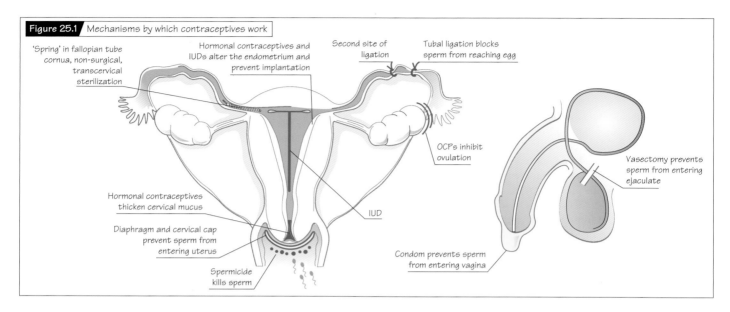

Figure 25.1 Mechanisms by which contraceptives work

'Spring' in fallopian tube cornua, non-surgical, transcervical sterilization

Hormonal contraceptives and IUDs alter the endometrium and prevent implantation

Second site of ligation

Tubal ligation blocks sperm from reaching egg

OCPs inhibit ovulation

Vasectomy prevents sperm from entering ejaculate

Hormonal contraceptives thicken cervical mucus

IUD

Diaphragm and cervical cap prevent sperm from entering uterus

Spermicide kills sperm

Condom prevents sperm from entering vagina

The risk of pregnancy without contraception is 2–4% for each unprotected act of intercourse. In 100 women using no contraception, 85 pregnancies occur per year. Approximately half of all pregnancies in the developed world are unplanned and many of these women report using some form of reversible birth control at the time they became pregnant. Only absolute abstinence completely prevents pregnancy. While no form of contraception is perfect in sexually active women, helping patients to choose a contraceptive method that they are able to use consistently and correctly can decrease unintended pregnancy (Fig. 25.1). With perfect use, oral contraceptives (OC) are nearly as effective as long-acting reversible contraceptives (LARC), such as the intrauterine device (IUD), progesterone intramuscular injection and progesterone implants. However, with typical use, LARC methods are approximately 10 times more effective.

"Natural" family planning

Natural family planning or fertility awareness aims to avoid conception by abstention from intercourse during the woman's fertile period. It makes use of a calendar and some indicator of ovulation (basal body temperature measurements, cervical mucus characteristics or commercial ovulation prediction kits). Intercourse is avoided during the so-called fertile period at ovulation and for several days before and after. Natural family planning requires a highly motivated couple, regular menstrual cycles and the willingness to tolerate a failure rate of up to 25%. The method has no medical side effects and is accepted by virtually all religions.

Barrier methods

There are three general categories of barrier contraception: condom, diaphragm and cervical cap. All work by preventing spermatozoa from entering the woman's uterus and fertilizing an egg. Barrier methods are good choices for individuals who want to limit contraceptive efficacy to a particular sexual episode. They are readily reversible and can be used in conjunction with the timing methods associated with natural family planning. The most serious side effects of barrier methods occur in individuals with an unknown latex allergy.

Condoms that fit over the penis are more widely available than condoms that fit inside the vagina (the female condom). Male condoms may be made from latex rubber, polyurethane or animal intestines; each provides a different "feel" or sensitivity for the man during intercourse. Female condoms are typically made of polyurethane. Intact condoms stop sperm and infectious agents from entering the vagina and so can prevent transmission of HIV and other sexually transmitted diseases. They must be carefully removed after ejaculation to avoid spilling semen from the condom into the vagina. The failure rates of condoms are 3–6% with perfect use and 15% with typical use.

The **diaphragm** is a soft latex or plastic dome that fits inside the vagina and covers the cervix. Because some sperm may be able to bypass the diaphragm and gain access to the uterus, spermicide is placed in the dome of the diaphragm. Diaphragms are individually fitted by a clinician and require some training for proper insertion and removal. A diaphragm should be left in place for 6–8 h after intercourse, and additional spermicide placed into the vagina if more episodes of intercourse occur before it is removed. Diaphragms partially protect against HIV and other sexually transmitted diseases. Some women develop bladder or vaginal infections during diaphragm use. The failure rate of a properly fitted diaphragm with perfect use is about 6%; it rises to 15% with typical use.

Cervical caps are similar to, but smaller than, the diaphragm. They are individually fitted to tightly cover the cervix. Failure rates are similar to those of the diaphragm. Cervical caps are not widely available.

Spermicides

These are chemicals that kill sperm by disrupting their outer cell membranes. The most commonly used are nonoxynol-9 and octoxynol-9. Spermicides are available suspended in one of three vehicles: foam, jelly or wax suppositories. Spermacides are recommended for use with a barrier method, because the failure rate of spermicide used alone is up to 30%. There are few absolute contraindications to their use. They have an unpleasant taste and can cause an allergy in some

The Reproductive System at a Glance, Fourth Edition. Linda J. Heffner and Danny J. Schust.

users. Spermicide use may cause inflammation of the female genital tract and has been associated with an increase in the transmission of sexually transmitted infections, including HIV.

Intrauterine devices

The IUD is a small T-shaped device, placed into the uterine cavity and attached to a monofilament thread that hangs into the vagina, allowing the user to confirm that it remains in place. The modern IUD provides safe, long-acting, highly effective and rapidly reversible contraception with few side effects. The precise contraceptive mechanism of the IUD is not known, but it is thought to work by preventing fertilization as well as causing the endometrium to be inhospitable for implantation. The 10–12 year copper IUD produces a local inflammatory response in the endometrium and excess prostaglandin production. The copper ion competitively inhibits a number of zinc-requiring processes in sperm activation and endometrium/embryo signaling. The 3- and 5+-year progestin-releasing IUDs thickens cervical mucus, creating a barrier to sperm penetration into the upper genital tract. Additionally, the progestin disrupts the normal proliferative-to-secretory sequence of endometrial maturation.

Historically, IUDs, such as the Dalkon Shield, were associated with increased risk for medical complications and reproductive damage among users who were infected with sexually transmitted pathogens. This increased risk was likely due to the braided IUD tail, which allowed bacteria to ascend into the upper genital tract. The monofilament string, used on all modern IUDs, does not have this risk. In women at high risk for sexually transmitted infections (STIs), screening should be performed prior to IUD insertion. Women should be advised to use a barrier method for prevention of HIV and other STIs.

Side effects of the copper IUD include increased menstrual bleeding, iron-deficiency anemia and dysmenorrhea. The progestin IUD reduces menstrual flow and may be used to treat menorrhagia and adenomyosis. The IUD is highly effective, with a failure rate <1% per year. If pregnancy occurs, it is more likely to be ectopic in location. However, compared with women using no form of contraception, women with IUDs still have a reduced risk of ectopic pregnancy.

Hormonal contraception

Combination oral contraceptive pills (often called OCPs) are the most widely used form of hormonal contraception. They include a synthetic estrogen (ethinyl estradiol or mestranol) combined with a variety of synthetic progestins and are typically taken orally for 21 consecutive days of every 28 and allow monthly withdrawal bleeding. The progestin component of combination OCPs varies in its activity on progesterone receptors, androgen receptors and mineralocorticoid receptors. The estrogen and progestin dosages in monthly combination OCPs may be constant over the 21 days or may be sequentially modulated (phased or triphasic pills). Some newer combination oral contraceptive regimens provide continuous rather than monthly exogenous hormone cycles, often allowing endometrial sloughing only 3-4 times per year. Combination OCPs prevent pregnancy by multiple mechanisms, including inhibition of ovulation, thickening of cervical mucus to prevent sperm transport and alteration of the uterine lining to block implantation.

OCPs have benefits beyond pregnancy prevention, including decreased risk of pelvic inflammatory disease (PID), benign breast disease, anemia and endometrial and ovarian cancer. They are not totally risk free, however, and are associated with increased risk of thromboembolic disease, nonthrombotic stroke and gallbladder disease. Women over 35 who smoke should not use combination OCPs. Failure rates are <1% with perfect use and about 8% with typical use. To be effective, OCPs must be taken in the correct order on a daily basis.

Combinations of estrogen and progestin are also available for contraception in nonoral formulations. These include transdermal patches, injections and vaginal rings. All have efficacy similar to combination OCPs, and may have reduced metabolic side effect profiles.

Progestin-only contraceptives can be administered orally, by intramuscular injection or as a subdermal implant. All work by thickening cervical mucus and altering the endometrial lining of the uterus. The oral form of the progestin-only contraceptive, often called the mini-pill, is useful in women with contraindications to estrogen such as breastfeeding or high thrombotic risk. With perfect use, the mini-pill has a failure rate comparable with OCPs. However, the half-life of the mini-pill is short, with nearly undetectable plasma levels at 24 h. Thus, to maximize effectiveness, the mini-pill requires precise compliance with all 28 active pills taken at the same time daily.

Depo-medroxyprogesterone acetate (DMPA) is a progestin contraceptive given as an intramuscular injection every 12–14 weeks. Common side effects include irregular bleeding, particularly in the first 6 months of use, and weight gain. Because of the length of action of DMPA, side effects may persist until the medication is cleared and return to fertility may be delayed.

The original six-capsule subdermal levonorgestrel progestin implant (Norplant) has been replaced with an equivalent two-capsule system (Jadelle, 5 years of use), and a single capsule subdermal etonorgestrel implant (Implanon, 3 years of use). Insertion and removal are generally quick and uncomplicated, but must be performed by a trained clinician. Side effects include irregularly irregular vaginal bleeding.

Hormonal emergency contraception can be effective in preventing pregnancy if taken within the given time interval after unprotected intercourse or a contraceptive failure. Plan B, consisting of 1.5 mg levonorgestral, prevents pregnancy using the same mechanisms as other progestin contraceptives if taken within 120 h of exposure. Combination estrogen–progestin emergency contraception may also be used up to 120 h following exposure; however, the combined hormonal regimen has more side effects and a lower effectiveness than the progestin-only regimen. The copper IUD may also be used for emergency contraception up to 5 days after unprotected intercourse.

Sterilization

Sterilization of both men and women are surgical methods of permanent contraception. Sterilization prevents the gametes from reaching the point of fertilization.

In women, sterilization is commonly performed by laparoscopic **tubal ligation**. Tubal ligation interrupts the fallopian tubes and may involve the use of tying, blockade, cautery, partial excision or banding. Ten-year cumulative failure rates for female sterilization are 0.75–3.5%, depending upon the method. If a pregnancy does occur after tubal ligation, up to 50% are in an ectopic (tubal) location because of the blockage of the fallopian tube. **Transcervical sterilization** involves placement of micro-inserts into the fallopian tubes using a hysteroscope. This method requires no incision and can be performed in a doctor's office. Disadvantages include the need to wait 3 months for tubal occlusion to occur and confirmation of occlusion using a radiographic dye test called a hysterosalpingogram. Failure rates appear similar to laparoscopic methods.

The sterilization procedure used in men is called a **vasectomy**. It involves bilateral interruption of the vas deferens as they leave the testes in the scrotum. Surgical methods for interruption include partial excision, cautery or tying. Vasectomy is typically 100% effective but requires a 3-month waiting period and multiple postprocedure ejaculations to clear the vas deferens of previously produced sperm.

26 Abnormalities of male sexual differentiation and development

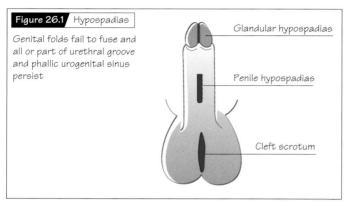

Figure 26.1 | Hypospadias

Genital folds fail to fuse and all or part of urethral groove and phallic urogenital sinus persist

Glandular hypospadias

Penile hypospadias

Cleft scrotum

Cryptorchidism

An undescended testis (cryptorchidism) is the most common genital abnormality seen in male newborn infants. It occurs in 3% of babies. Either one or both testes may be involved. Cryptorchidism occurs when the gubernaculum fails to develop or fails to pull the testes into the scrotum. Androgen activity directs gubernacular development and function, thus gubernacular dysfunction reflects androgen abnormalities. Insufficient androgen activity can result from developmental defects anywhere along the fetal hypothalamic–pituitary–testicular axis. To this point, cryptorchidism can result from any of the following: (i) fetal hypothalamic failure to stimulate gonadotropin secretion in the third trimester (Kallmann and Prader–Willi syndromes, anencephaly); (ii) failure of the testes to secrete androgens (gonadal dysgenesis); (iii) failure of testosterone conversion to dihydrotestosterone (DHT) in target tissues (5α-reductase deficiency); or (iv) absence of functioning androgen receptors (androgen insensitivity syndromes) (Table 26.1).

Cryptorchid testes may remain in the inguinal canal (70%), the abdomen or retroperitoneum (25%), or other ectopic locations (5%). Testes remaining in the abdomen or inguinal canal will be exposed to comparatively higher temperatures than those in the scrotum and will cease spermatogenesis in response. They are also prone to neoplastic change. Medical therapy for cryptorchidism involves administration of human chorionic gonadotropin (hCG) or androgens. Surgical therapy is called orchiopexy. Some cryptorchid testes are unresponsive to medications or cannot be brought into the scrotum surgically. These testes are usually removed because they cannot be adequately monitored for the development of a neoplasm.

Inguinal hernia is a forme fruste of cryptorchidism. Here, testicular descent occurs, but the inguinal ring does not close completely after descent. Boys who have an inguinal hernia diagnosed before the age of 15 have twice the risk of developing testicular cancer when compared to boys in the general population.

Hypospadias

Hypospadias is a very common congenital abnormality seen in male newborn infants. In hypospadias, the urethral meatus opens on to the ventral surface of the penile shaft at sites proximal to the normal location (Fig. 26.1). Embryologically, hypospadias results from a failure of complete ventral closure of the urethral groove. The penile urethra depends on the androgen DHT to differentiate. Therefore, hypospadias can result from deficiencies in testosterone (T) production, from inadequate conversion of T to DHT, or from local deficiencies in androgen recognition (insufficient androgen receptor number or function). There is a non-Mendelian genetic predisposition to hypospadias. If one sibling has a hypospadias, the recurrence risk is 12% in that family. If both the father and a brother are affected, the risk for a second son is 25%.

Cryptorchidism is seen in 16% of boys with hypospadias. If both are present, the child may be a pseudohermaphrodite and chromosomal and hormonal testing should be obtained.

Congenital bilateral absence of the vas deferens

Congenital bilateral absence of the vas deferens (CBAVD) is a rare congenital anomaly found most often in men with cystic fibrosis (CF). It can also occur in the absence of clinically apparent CF. When it does, it is usually associated with mutations in the gene coding for the CF transmembrane receptor (CFTR). The molecular mechanism by which an abnormal transmembrane receptor involved in chloride channels leads either to failure of the vas deferens to differentiate or to its resorption is not known. The presence of CBAVD mandates genetic testing for CF genes.

Microorchidism

The presence of at least one additional X chromosome in most of the cells of a man with Kleinfelter syndrome (usually 47XXY) results in hypogonadism and frequent infertility and microorchidism. XXY men are variably affected with other physical (tall stature, gynecomastia) and behavioral (speech and learning) problems. This is the most common sex chromosome aneuploidy in males and may be one of the most common chromosome abnormalities in humans.

Pseudohermaphroditism

Individuals possessing testes, but in the presence of external and/or internal genitalia with a female phenotype are called male pseudohermaphrodites. Gonadal sex does not match genital phenotype. Male pseudohermaphroditism results from an inappropriate fetal hormonal environment. This can be caused by biochemical defects in androgen activity or by abnormal sex chromosome constitution. Pseudohermaphroditism is a rare disorder, but its multiple etiologies have offered the opportunity to further understand the role of steroids in human genital development. A list of the known biochemical defects leading to male pseudohermaphroditism includes:

- Androgen insensitivity syndromes
- 5α-reductase deficiency
- Testosterone biosynthesis defects
- Congenital adrenal hyperplasia (CAH) syndromes
- Impaired androgenization
- Anti-Müllerian hormone defect.

Androgen insensitivity syndromes

The androgen insensitivity syndromes are a group of X-linked recessive traits that produce a spectrum of incompletely virilized phenotypes. The most severe form, **complete androgen insensitivity (AI)**, was originally known as **testicular feminization**. In complete AI, the intracellular androgen receptor is absent or nonfunctional. Androgen induction of Wolffian duct development does not occur. Müllerian-inhibiting substance (MIS) is produced by the normally functioning testes and the Müllerian ducts regress. The testes descend to the level of the inguinal ring under the influence of MIS. A short vagina forms

The Reproductive System at a Glance, Fourth Edition. Linda J. Heffner and Danny J. Schust.

60 © 2014 John Wiley & Sons, Ltd. Published 2014 by John Wiley & Sons, Ltd. Companion Website: www.ataglanceseries.com/reproduction

from the urogenital sinus. At birth, children with complete AI are typically assigned the female sex because there is no trace of androgen activity and the external genitalia clearly appear female. Complete AI is typically diagnosed after puberty when primary amenorrhea becomes apparent. Examination of the complete AI individual reveals a blind-ending, short vagina and an absent cervix, uterus and ovaries. Breast development is normal, but axillary and pubic hair is scant or absent. Complete AI accounts for about 10% of all cases of primary amenorrhea. In contrast to those individuals with a dysgenetic gonad bearing a Y chromosome, those with complete AI have less than a 5% risk of developing a gonadal tumor. Gonadal tumors that do develop in AI patients rarely appear before age 25. Therefore, gonadectomy is postponed until puberty is complete.

The **incomplete androgen insensitivity syndrome (Reifenstein syndrome)** is far less common than the complete and is associated with a broad spectrum of phenotypes. These vary from almost complete failure of internal and external genital virilization to complete phenotypic masculinization. Between these extremes exist patients with mild clitoromegaly and slight labial fusion to those with significant genital ambiguity. Recently, several men have been described whose only indication of AI was infertility resulting from low or absent sperm production. Some fertile males who appear undervirilized probably have a mild form of this disorder.

Incomplete AI results from mutations in the androgen receptor gene. The gene encoding the androgen receptor localizes to the q11-12 region of the X chromosome. Defects can occur in the androgen-binding domain of the receptor, the DNA-binding domain of the receptor or in receptor protein production. Identified abnormalities range from complete loss of receptor function to subtle qualitative changes in the transcription of androgen-dependent target genes. There is poor correlation between absolute androgen receptor levels and the degree of masculinization seen in patients with incomplete AI.

5α-reductase deficiency

The syndrome seen among patients with 5α-reductase deficiency was originally given the name **pseudovaginal perineoscrotal hypospadias (PPH)**. It differs from AI in that masculinization occurs at puberty. At birth, individuals with 5α-reductase deficiency have external genitalia that resemble those of incomplete AI, including hypospadias, varying degrees of failure of the labioscrotal folds to fuse and either a urogenital opening or separate vaginal and urethral openings. The cleft in the scrotum resembles a vagina and most children with 5α-reductase deficiency are raised as girls. In these patients, adrenal steroid production is normal and the karyotype is XY. Measuring blood levels of testosterone and DHT and demonstrating an elevated T:DHT ratio can establish the diagnosis of 5α-reductase deficiency and eliminate the diagnosis of CAH in an incompletely virilized newborn infant (Chapter 27).

Molecular analyses have demonstrated that there are two 5α-reductase genes; mutations in the isoenzyme coded on chromosome 2 (*SRD5A2* gene) are responsible for this form of male pseudo-hermaphroditism. Multiple mutations of *SRD5A2* have been identified. The segregation of the same specific defects in unrelated individuals of the same ethnicity suggests common ancestry. Compound heterozygotes are common, suggesting that the gene frequency for *SRD5A2* mutations may be fairly high. Women are not clinically affected by 5α-reductase deficiency.

Congenital adrenal hyperplasia syndromes

A group of enzymatic defects of the steroidogenic pathways cause reproductive and metabolic disorders collectively known as the CAH syndromes. Among these, **lipoid congenital adrenal hyperplasia (StAR protein deficiency), 3β-hydroxysteroid dehydrogenase deficiency, 17α-hydroxylase deficiency and 17β-hydroxysteroid dehydrogenase deficiency** can cause feminization of fetal external genitalia. All are specific enzymatic defects in the steroidogenic pathway common to the testes and adrenal glands and all involve enzymes occurring early in the steroidogenic pathway between cholesterol and testosterone (Chapters 2 and 29). CAH syndromes that cause masculinization in female fetuses are much more common and result from enzymatic defects more distal in the steroidogenic pathways.

Gender assignment

Gender assignment in male infants with pseudohermaphroditism requires knowledge of the specific defect. Most are raised as females. Individuals with complete AI (testicular feminization) are raised as females because they unambiguously appear as females at birth. In addition, because they lack functional androgen receptors, AI patients will never be virilized. Males whose incomplete AI presents with ambiguous genitalia are also usually raised as females because predictable feminization with gynecomastia will occur at puberty. Males with 5α-reductase deficiency have been successfully raised as either females or males. In fact, in cultures with a high frequency of the disorder, children have been raised as females in childhood and males after puberty. Patients with 5α-reductase deficiency who are assigned as females and wish to retain their female gender will need to be gonadectomized to avoid deepening of their voices and a male pattern of muscle development that will occur at puberty. Both will occur in response to pubertal testosterone, a substance to which they can respond. Estrogen and progesterone therapy can be used to produce female secondary sexual development. Patients with 5α-reductase deficiency who are assigned to the male gender require repair of their hypospadias and cryptorchidism. At puberty, spermatogenesis and masculine sexual maturation will occur under the influence of testosterone.

True gonadal dysgenesis is relatively rare in individuals with an XY karyotype. Bilateral dysgenesis of the testes (**Swyer syndrome**) results in normal, but infantile female external and internal genital development and lack of secondary sexual development at puberty. Fibrous bands appear in place of the testes. Gonadectomy is necessary to prevent the 20–30% risk of tumor formation. Estrogen and progesterone therapy support female secondary sexual development at puberty.

Table 26.1 The androgen insensitivity syndromes

	Complete	Reifenstein	Infertile	5α-reductase
Inheritance	X-linked recessive	X-linked recessive	X-linked recessive	Autosomal recessive
Spermatogenesis	Absent	Absent	Decreased	Decreased
Müllerian structures	Absent	Absent	Absent	Absent
Wolffian structures	Absent	Male	Male	Male
External genitalia	Female	Male/hypospadias	Male	Female
Breasts (puberty)	Female	Female/gynecomastia	Gynecomastia	Male

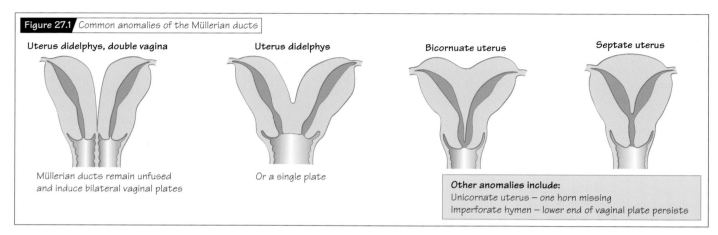

Figure 27.1 Common anomalies of the Müllerian ducts

Uterus didelphys, double vagina

Müllerian ducts remain unfused and induce bilateral vaginal plates

Uterus didelphys

Or a single plate

Bicornuate uterus

Septate uterus

Other anomalies include:
Unicornate uterus – one horn missing
Imperforate hymen – lower end of vaginal plate persists

Structural anomalies

Structural anomalies of the uterus, cervix and vagina are the most common abnormalities of sexual differentiation seen in women. They arise from embryologic abnormalities of Müllerian system development (Chapters 5 and 6). The most severe form involves complete absence of the reproductive tract, including the vagina, uterus and fallopian tubes. Such agenesis of the Müllerian system is known as Mayer–Rokitansky–Kuster–Hauser syndrome, and is the second most common cause of primary amenorrhea (Chapter 30).

The remainder of the anomalies result from failure of the Müllerian system to fuse in the midline or to remodel in the midline after fusion to form a single uterine cavity (Fig. 27.1). The most dramatic form of fusion anomalies occurs when the Müllerian ducts fail to fuse along their entire length, resulting in the formation of two vaginas, two cervices and two separate uterine horns (double uterus or *uterus didelphys*). More commonly, only the upper portion of the uterus fails to fuse. The uterine body may then remain separated as two horns (bicornuate uterus or *uterus bicornus*) or, in milder cases, a dimple may be noted in the contour of the uterine fundus (arcuate uterus). Occasionally, only one side of the Müllerian system will develop, resulting in a hemi-uterus and a single fallopian tube (unicornuate uterus or *uterus unicornus*).

Failure to resorb the midline of the Müllerian ducts after fusion typically results in a uterine septum. A septum may be complete, running from the cervix to the fundus, or incomplete, involving only the uterine fundus (subseptate uterus). Occasionally, the vagina canalizes improperly and a vaginal septum will occur. This can occur in isolation or in conjunction with a uterine anomaly. Vaginal septa can be either longitudinal or horizontal. The longitudinal septum is reminiscent of those uterine anomalies resulting from failure of the Müllerian midline to resorb. Horizontal vaginal septa are thought to represent a failure of the vaginal plate to resorb at the site where it fuses with the Müllerian ducts.

Many women with structural anomalies of the reproductive tract are asymptomatic and never diagnosed. Others with Müllerian tract abnormalities may present with primary amenorrhea, recurrent miscarriages, preterm delivery and breech presentation at term. **Because the mesonephros is closely involved in directing the development of the internal genitalia, the finding of a uterine anomaly should prompt an evaluation of the urinary system for an accompanying anomaly.**

Exposure to diethylstilbestrol

In utero exposure to diethylstilbestrol (DES) occurred in individuals born between 1940 and 1971 whose mothers were given the synthetic estrogen in the hope of preventing a miscarriage. DES was subsequently shown to cause congenital abnormalities in women and, to a lesser degree, in men. The most frequently seen abnormalities in women are abnormally shaped cervices. These cervices have been described as coxcomb, hooded or hypoplastic. The uterine musculature may also be abnormally formed in DES-exposed women such that the uterine cavity assumes a T-shape on hysterosalpingography or saline-infusion sonohysterography. DES appears to cause these abnormalities via inappropriate activation of estrogen-dependent genes involved in differentiating the cervix and upper third of the vagina from the lower vagina. This results not only in the structurally abnormal cervices and uteri, but also in persistence of cervical glandular epithelium in the vagina (**vaginal adenosis**). *In utero* DES exposure is associated with an increased risk of reproductive failure, including infertility (likely from failed implantation), recurrent pregnancy loss and preterm delivery. DES daughters are also at increased risk for malignancies, specifically clear cell adenocarcinoma, arising in sites of vaginal adenosis. This is thought to result from exposure of the ectopic cervical glandular-type epithelia in the vagina to neoplastic inducers not usually accessible to the upper reproductive tract.

Occasionally, clinicians will observe cervical and uterine abnormalities that look exactly like those caused by *in utero* DES exposure in women never exposed to DES.

Congenital adrenal hyperplasia

Ambiguous genitalia in a newborn infant are most commonly caused by congenital adrenal hyperplasia (CAH). This diagnosis accounts for 40–50% of all cases of ambiguous genitalia. Depending on the degree of the defect and the particular steroidogenic enzyme that is dysfunctional, neonatal effects can be variable. Affected female infants may have a common urogenital sinus containing the vagina and urethra, which opens at the base of an enlarged phallus resembling a penis. The labia majora may be hypertrophied or fused and thus resemble an empty scrotum. Some female infants will appear like a male with hypospadias and cryptorchidism. Others will only exhibit mild to moderate clitoromegaly. Some of these infants will have accompany-

Table 27.1 "Virilizing" forms of congenital adrenal hyperplasia (see Fig. 2.1)

Enzyme deficiency	Clinical appearance	Cortisol	Aldosterone	Androgens
21β-hydroxylase – severe	Salt-wasting, virilized	–	–	++
21β-hydroxylase – moderate	Virilized	Normal	+	++
21β-hydroxylase – mild	Adult polycystic ovaries	Normal	+/–	+
11β-hydroxylase	Hypertensive, virilized	–	–	++
17α-hydroxylase	Hypertensive	–	+/–	–

ing hypertension (5%) or life-threatening salt wasting (30%) and this will aid in making the diagnosis soon after birth. Those carrying the most common defect, moderate 21β-hydroxylase deficiency, will have no other identifying characteristics. **The finding of a normal female karyotype in a newborn assigned to the male gender in the delivery room requires an evaluation for CAH.**

The primary defect in all types of CAH is the absence of one of the enzymes necessary for steroidogenesis. The most common forms involve the enzymes that convert androgens to the adrenal steroids (Table 27.1). In the absence of one of these enzymes, no steroidal end-product will be produced by the adrenal gland to feed back on the hypothalamic–pituitary axis and regulate adrenocorticotropic hormone (ACTH) secretion. Excess ACTH will continue to stimulate the adrenals to produce more of the steroid products prior to the enzymatic block. These products are then shunted toward androgen-forming pathways. Adrenal hyperplasia with excess androgen production will result. This is of little consequence in the male fetus but will result in masculinization of the androgen-sensitive external genitalia in a female fetus. Because the female fetus has neither testes nor Müllerian-inhibiting substance (MIS), females affected by CAH will have uteri and vaginas. The degree of hypertrophy and fusion of the external genitalia in CAH females will depend on the quantity of androgen involved and on the developmental timing of androgen exposure. Masculinized infants with ovaries and a 46XX karyotype are called female pseudohermaphrodites.

Therapy for **female infants masculinized as a result of CAH** includes glucocorticoid administration to suppress adrenal androgen secretion and genital reconstructive surgery. Infants who also have a defect in aldosterone synthesis will also require mineralocorticoid replacement.

Virilization of female infants by maternal or exogenous androgen exposure occurs only when those androgens are unable to be converted to estrogens by placental aromatase. Therefore, infants born to mothers with CAH are not at risk unless the child has inherited the genetic defect from both parents and also carries the enzymatic deficiency. Infants born to mothers with an androgen-producing tumor may be virilized if the particular androgen produced cannot be aromatized (e.g., dihydrotestosterone, DHT) or it quantitatively exceeds the high aromatization capacity of the placenta. Maternal administration of synthetic progestins with androgenic activity has also been associated with virilization of the female neonate; use of synthetic progesterones is contraindicated in pregnant women. Female virilization that has resulted from *in utero* steroid exposure but has no accompanying risk for postnatal exposure can be treated with reconstructive surgery alone.

Turner syndrome

Women with Turner syndrome are often identified when the physical characteristics of short stature, webbed neck, shield chest and increased carrying angle accompany primary amenorrhea. The fundamental defect in Turner syndrome patients is the absence of a second sex chromosome(i.e., a 45X karyotype). In the absence of a functional second sex chromosome, the germ cells in the gonad do not survive past the embryonic period and a normal ovary or testis does not develop. Gonadal steroid synthesis and secretion do not occur during embryogenesis or at puberty. Systems other than reproduction are affected by Turner syndrome. Women with the disorder have an increased incidence of renal anomalies, autoimmune diseases and cardiac anomalies, particularly coarctation of the aorta and aortic aneurysms. Turner syndrome is the most common of a group of disorders known as **gonadal dysgenesis**.

Most individuals with gonadal dysgenesis have a female phenotype at birth. If the entirety of the second sex chromosome is missing, both the external and internal genitalia will be female. After puberty, these female structures will remain infantile because of the lack of ovarian estrogens from the nonfunctional gonad. If any remnant of a second sex chromosome is present in an individual with gonadal dysgenesis, the phenotype will depend on the specific genes retained. For instance, if the SRY locus is present and translocated onto another chromosome, signals to begin testicular differentiation will occur. MIS will be produced and the Müllerian duct system will regress. Despite MIS production, these individuals will have a rudimentary testis and lack androgen production. They will be born with female external genitalia, but lack a vagina and other female internal reproductive structures. Primordial Wolffian ducts may be identified at laparotomy along with ovotestes. These rare individuals are **true hermaphrodites**.

Sex chromosome **mosaicism** (multiple cell lines of different sex chromosomal composition) is not uncommon in Turner syndrome. Individuals carrying any portion of the Y chromosome, including SRY alone, may have a testicular component to their dysgenetic gonad. These patients are at risk for gonadal malignancies and may have functional testicular tissue that causes virilization at puberty. Therefore it is important to confirm any suspected diagnosis of Turner syndrome using karyotype analysis. Some experts recommend using a DNA probe against SRY as well. Individuals who possess a cell line containing a Y chromosome or who carry SRY should undergo bilateral gonadectomy prior to puberty to eliminate the possibility of virilization or cancer.

If sex chromosome mosaicism involves a second X chromosome, functional ovarian tissue may exist within the gonad. Women with such mosaicism may experience normal female puberty and even retain fertility for a brief period of time. Early menopause invariably occurs because the abnormal chromosomal constitution causes development of only a limited number of functional ovarian follicles. A woman with complete Turner syndrome or XX mosaicism can carry a pregnancy conceived through *in vitro* fertilization using donated oocytes. Her infantile uterus will require extensive hormonal priming.

Sexual precocity is defined as the appearance of secondary sexual characteristics before the age of 8 years in girls and before the age of 9 years in boys. Recent data suggest that these ages are less than two standard deviations from the mean. Still, the ramifications of misdiagnosis are great and, at present, breast or pubic hair development before age 8 or menarche before age 10 warrants an evaluation in girls. Testicular enlargement or pubic hair development before age 9 in boys warrants similar investigation. While the appearance of all secondary sex characteristics results from increased sex steroid production, the underlying etiology of elevated sex hormone production and activity may be increased gonadotropin secretion or intrinsic disease of the adrenal, ovary or testis (Table 28.1). **Complete or true sexual precocity** is used to describe precocious puberty resulting from elevated pituitary gonadotropins. **Incomplete or peripheral sexual precocity** refers to precocious puberty resulting from primary diseases of the gonads or adrenals. Early sexual development that is consistent with the genetic and gonadal sex of the individual is **isosexual precocity**. **Heterosexual** or **contrasexual precocity** indicates precocious puberty associated with feminization of a male or virilization of a female.

Although more than half the cases of isosexual precocious puberty simply represent the early end of the normal developmental spectrum, all children with sexual precocity should be evaluated. There are several reasons for this recommendation. First, some children may have a serious disorder associated with precocious puberty. Second, regardless of the etiology, sexual development that occurs before age 6–7 years can be associated with short stature in adulthood if left untreated. An X-ray of the left wrist to evaluate **bone age** can be used to determine when to initiate and stop chosen treatments for precocious puberty and to follow treatment efficacy. Finally, **sexual precocity is not accompanied by advanced psychosexual maturation**. To this point, young girls with precocious puberty appear to be at significant risk for sexual abuse. Ovulation and conception are possible and pregnancies in girls as young as 5 years of age have occurred as the result of such abuse. Appropriate therapy and support are necessary to prevent the potential long-term consequences of sexual precocity.

True or complete precocious puberty

True sexual precocity results from early maturation of the hypothalamic–pituitary–gonadal (HPG) axis. Measurements of serum gonadotropins and sex steroid concentrations will be in the normal postpubertal range. Gonadotropin pulsatility will have characteristics and feedback regulation similar to those found in the adult. The physical characteristics of puberty appear prematurely, but in the proper chronologic order. One half of cases of true sexual precocity arise from premature activation of the HPG axis (Table 28.2).

The remaining cases of complete isosexual precocity are caused by central nervous system (CNS) lesions. These lesions include neoplasms, trauma, hydrocephalus, postinfectious encephalitis, congenital brain defects, tuberous sclerosis and neurofibromatosis type 1. Most lesions are located in, or near, the posterior hypothalamus. The most commonly identified neoplasms are astrocytomas, ependymomas and craniopharyngiomas. Hamartomas of the tuber cinereum account for one in six cases of isosexual precocious puberty in girls and half of the cases in boys. Hamartomas are congenital malformations that contain fibre bundles, glial cells and gonadotropin-releasing hormone (GnRH)-secreting neurons.

Although a rare cause of precocious puberty, girls with severe primary hypothyroidism can develop hyperprolactinemia, associated galactorrhea and true precocious puberty. These girls have a primary defect in the thyroid gland and very high thyroid-stimulating hormone (TSH) levels in response to low thyroid hormone secretion. They also have elevated circulating gonadotropins. The development of precocious puberty in girls with primary hypothyroidism may be the result of gonadotropin stimulation of the ovary, or from cross-activation of the follicle-stimulating hormone (FSH) receptor by the pathologically high TSH. In the face of low thyroid hormone secretion, hypothalamic thyrotropin-releasing hormone (TRH) production rises. TRH is a potent stimulator of prolactin secretion by pituitary lactotrophs (Chapter 32); hyperprolactinemia and galactorrhea result.

Occasionally, the development of true sexual precocity will follow the correction of a long-standing virilizing condition in girls. This may occur with treatment of congenital adrenal hyperplasia (CAH). Correction of excess androgen production releases the hypothalamus from androgen-associated negative feedback. This permits GnRH secretion and gonadotropin stimulation of the ovary. The timing of this stimulation may be inappropriate and, in a young girl, lead to complete precocious isosexual development.

Treatment of true precocious puberty involves recognition and correction of underlying CNS lesions if etiologic. Additional therapy may be required, including suppression of the HPG axis with a GnRH agonist or antagonist. GnRH agonists are long-acting analogs of GnRH that occupy its receptors for long periods of time. Prolonged receptor occupation removes the GnRH pulsatility required for appropriate gonadotropin release from the pituitary. GnRH antagonists occupy and block GnRH receptors and cause immediate cessation of GnRH pulsatility. Both are effective in protecting adult height and avoiding many psychosexual issues surrounding untreated precocious puberty.

Incomplete isosexual precocity

Incomplete isosexual precocity is caused by ovarian or adrenal secretion of estrogen in girls and testicular or adrenal secretion of androgen in boys. In girls, the most common cause of GnRH-independent precocious puberty is the presence of functionally autonomous ovarian cysts. Small (<1 cm) follicles occur frequently in the prepubertal ovary but they rarely secrete significant amounts of estrogen. However, autonomous secretion of estradiol by the granulosa cells contained in the cyst wall can occur in larger cysts, and serum estradiol concentrations appear to correlate directly with cyst size. Progestin therapy can reduce the size of these cysts and prevent their recurrence.

Solid stromal cell tumors of the ovary are a rare cause of GnRH-independent precocious puberty in girls. When compared with functional cysts of the ovary, juvenile granulosa or theca cell tumors secrete very large amounts of estrogen, often resulting in the rapid development of sexual characteristics.

Two inherited syndromes, Peutz–Jeghers and McCune–Albright, are associated with isosexual precocious puberty. Peutz–Jeghers syndrome is defined by the appearance of mucocutaneous pigmentation and gastrointestinal polyposis, but may also include gonadal sex cord tumors. McCune–Albright syndrome is characterized by hyperpigmented café-au-lait spots on the skin, progressive polyostotic fibrous dysplasia of the bones and GnRH-independent sexual precocity. Hyperplasia or adenomas of multiple endocrine glands may also occur.

The Reproductive System at a Glance, Fourth Edition. Linda J. Heffner and Danny J. Schust.

64 © 2014 John Wiley & Sons, Ltd. Published 2014 by John Wiley & Sons, Ltd. Companion Website: www.ataglanceseries.com/reproduction

McCune–Albright syndrome is caused by activating mutations in a signal transduction protein linked to many of the peptide hormone receptors, the G-protein subunit, $G_s\alpha$. These proteins are present in many cells and therefore many tissues can be affected; distribution may be patchy and unpredictable because mutations occur in postzygotic somatic cells. In girls with McCune–Albright syndrome and ovarian involvement, sexual precocity occurs because of estrogen secretion from luteinized follicular cysts and treatment involves interruption of estrogen production. CNS involvement is unlikely and patients with McCune–Albright syndrome can progress normally through GnRH-dependent puberty.

Incomplete isosexual precocious puberty is rare in boys. It is always caused by excess androgen exposure. Adrenal sources of androgen exposure include CAH and adrenal adenomas or cancers. Most virilizing adrenal tumors in children secrete excess amounts of dehydroepiandrosterone sulfate (DHEA-S). The DHEA-S, in turn, is converted to more potent androgens (Chapter 2). Testicular sources of androgen excess include Leydig cell tumors. These rare tumors of the testis produce testosterone.

Iatrogenic sexual precocity

Breast development has been reported in girls and boys after exposure to exogenous estrogens found in tonics, lotions, creams and estrogen-contaminated meat. Virilization of boys and girls has been associated with exposure to androgenic steroid preparations.

Virilizing precocious puberty in girls

Most girls with contrasexual precocious puberty will develop pubic hair or hirsutism. The most common cause is CAH. CAH is associated with multiple defects in the steroid synthetic pathway. Mild alterations in adrenal 21-hydroxylase are present in 0.1–1.0% of the population. These alterations may not manifest themselves as early as those of classical CAH; mild deficiencies are associated with late virilization, premature adrenarche, polycystic ovarian disease and postpubertal oligoamenorrhea. Diagnosis of this disorder rests on the presence of mild baseline elevations in 17-hydroxyprogesterone, the steroid precursor metabolized by 21-hydroxylase. Some patients with CAH will be discovered only after provocative testing, characterized by the exaggerated release of 17-hydroxyprogesterone to adrenocorticotropic hormone (ACTH) stimulation. Deficiencies in 11β-hydroxylase deficiency or 3β-hydroxysteroid dehydrogenase can cause virilizing precocious puberty in girls, but occur rarely.

Virilizing adrenal tumors that occur in young girls are very aggressive and usually fatal if malignant. Ovarian Leydig cell and Sertoli cell tumors are the most common virilizing neoplasms in women. They are a rare cause of virilizing precocious puberty.

Feminizing precocious puberty in boys

Contrasexual precocity is much less common in boys than in girls. Boys with feminizing precocious puberty will exhibit gynecomastia and accelerated linear bone growth. The presence of prepubertal-size testes on examination strongly suggests an adrenal or testicular source for the estrogen. One rare cause of prepubertal feminization is extraglandular aromatization of androstenedione. Gynecomastia has occasionally been seen with CAH in boys. Feminizing testicular tumors have been reported in boys with Peutz–Jeghers syndrome.

Table 28.1 Classification of precocious puberty

*Complete isosexual precocity (true precocious puberty –
    gonadotropin dependent)*
Idiopathic
CNS lesions
    Hamartomas
    Craniopharyngioma
Primary hypothyroidism
Following treatment for virilizing disorders in girls

Incomplete isosexual precocity (GnRH independent)
Estrogen-secreting neoplasms of ovary or adrenal in girls
Ovarian cysts
Androgen-secreting neoplasms of testis or adrenal in boys
McCune–Albright syndrome
Peutz–Jeghers syndrome

Iatrogenic sexual precocity

Contrasexual precocity
Virilization in females
    Congenital adrenal hyperplasia
    21-hydroxylase deficiency
    11β-hydroxylase deficiency
    3β-hydroxysteroid dehydrogenase deficiency
    Androgen-secreting ovarian or adrenal neoplasms
Feminization in males
Estrogen-secreting adrenal neoplasms

Table 28.2 Differential diagnosis of isosexual precocious puberty

	Serum gonadotropin concentration	LH response to GnRH	Serum sex steroid concentrations	Gonadal size	Miscellaneous
True precocious puberty (premature activation of hypothalamic GnRH pulse generator)	Prominent LH pulses	Pubertal LH response	Pubertal	Normal pubertal	MRI scan to rule out CNS abnormality, bone scan to exclude McCune–Albright syndrome
Incomplete sexual precocity (GnRH independent) Girls					
Follicular cysts	Low	Suppressed	Varies	Ovarian enlargement	Exclude McCune–Albright syndrome
Granulosa cell tumor	Low	Suppressed	Very high estradiol	Ovarian enlargement	Tumor may be palpable
Feminizing adrenal tumor	Low	Suppressed	High estradiol and DHEA-S	Prepubertal ovaries	Unilateral adrenal mass
Boys					
Congenital adrenal hyperplasia	Low	Suppressed	High 17-hydroxyprogesterone	Prepubertal testes	
Virilizing adrenal tumors	Low	Suppressed	High DHEA-S	Prepubertal	Unilateral adrenal mass
Leydig/Sertoli cell tumor	Low	Suppressed	High testosterone	Testicular mass	

DHEA-S, dehydroepiandrosterone sulfate; GnRH, gonadotropin-releasing hormone; LH, luteinizing hormone; MRI, magnetic resonance imaging.

Delayed puberty is defined as the absence of secondary sexual characteristics at age 13 in girls and 16 in boys (Chapters 11 and 12). It may result from: (i) a nonpathologic **constitutional delay** accompanying a growth delay; (ii) disorders of the hypothalamus or pituitary gland that result in inadequate gonadotropin secretion (**hypogonadotropic hypogonadism**); and (iii) disorders of the gonads that prevent adequate sex steroid secretion (**hypergonadotropic hypogonadism**) (Table 29.1). In girls, secondary sexual characteristics may develop without progression to menarche. This form of pubertal dysfunction and other causes of primary amenorrhoea are discussed in Chapter 30.

It is important to diagnose and treat delayed or absent puberty because: (i) serious underlying conditions may be present; (ii) abnormal persistence of a child-like phenotype has profound social implications for the teenager and young adult; (iii) prolonged absence of gonadal steroid exposure leads to osteopenia, a failure of normal bone formation. Osteopenia is associated with an increased risk of fractures in weight-bearing bones such as vertebrae, hips and long bones. Treatment of delayed or absent puberty aims to correct underlying disorders. Hormone replacement with estrogen/progesterone or testosterone is often required if hypogonadism is prolonged or age-appropriate sex steroid secretion patterns cannot be restored.

Constitutional pubertal delay

Pathologic causes of delayed puberty must be excluded before the diagnosis of constitutional pubertal delay can be considered. Constitutional pubertal delay is characterized by linear growth velocities and gonadotropin-releasing hormone (GnRH) secretory patterns that are appropriate for the individual's **bone age**. In girls, it has been observed that puberty begins at a bone age of 12 years. Therefore, a 13-year-old girl who has a bone age of 11 and has not developed secondary sexual characteristics may have constitutional delay.

Hypogonadotropic hypogonadism

This is characterized by **deficiencies in pulsatile GnRH, follicle-stimulating hormone (FSH) or luteinizing hormone (LH) secretion** that result in sexual infantilism. GnRH deficiencies arise via three general mechanisms: genetic defects of the hypothalamus, developmental defects of the hypothalamus and destructive lesions involving the hypothalamus or pituitary stalk.

The best characterized and most common of the genetic defects producing hypogonadotropic hypogonadism is **Kallmann syndrome**, which is typified by GnRH deficiency associated with hyposmia and hypoplasia of the olfactory lobes of the brain. It is inherited either as an X-linked recessive trait or as an autosomal dominant trait with variable penetrance. Kallmann syndrome is much more common in boys than in girls. Half of patients with Kallmann syndrome have mutations in the *KAL* gene on chromosome Xp22.3. This gene encodes an extracellular matrix protein that regulates axonal pathfinding and cellular adhesion. Deficiencies in the amounts, or function, of this protein explain the cluster of abnormalities associated with Kallmann syndrome: fetal GnRH neurosecretory neurons fail to migrate normally from the olfactory placode to the medial basal hypothalamus, resulting in inappropriate olfactory bulb development, anosmia and GnRH deficiencies.

Less common developmental defects have been associated with delayed or absent puberty due to hypogonadotropic hypogonadism. These also affect midline central nervous system (CNS) development.

Some have been described in association with visual abnormalities that result from developmental abnormalities in the optic tracts. GnRH deficiencies are often associated with other hypothalamic–pituitary functional abnormalities. As a result, delayed puberty is typically accompanied by short stature [growth hormone (GH) deficiency]. This can make differentiation from constitutional delay challenging. A familial form of isolated gonadotropin deficiency has also been described. Unlike most other forms of hypogonadotropic hypogonadism in which GH is also deficient, patients with familial isolated gonadotropin deficiency have normal height for bone age.

CNS tumors result in delayed puberty more often than precocious puberty. Most neoplasms that interfere with pubertal development are extrasellar and inhibit the production, or delivery, of the pituitary trophic hormones to the pituitary gland. Deficiencies in multiple pituitary hormones are common. Of these tumors, craniopharyngiomas are the most common cause of delayed or absent puberty. They originate from cells within the developmental anlagen of the anterior pituitary–Rathke's pouch, and are almost always located in or near the hypothalamus or pituitary. Many pituitary tumors that are common in adults are notably rare in prepubertal children. One, the prolactin-secreting adenomas, may occur among teenagers. Girls with prolactin-secreting pituitary adenomas may present to medical providers complaining of primary amenorrhea in the presence of secondary sexual characteristics. Neurofibromas of the CNS that develop as part of von Recklinghausen syndrome (neurofibromatosis) and germ-cell tumors can also be associated with sexual infantilism.

Functional gonadotropin deficiencies can arise from malnutrition, psychiatric disorders and from a large array of chronic diseases. Girls seem more sensitive than boys to the effects of malnutrition. In girls, a reduction to less than 80% of ideal body weight can be associated with delayed or arrested puberty. By contrast, starvation of famine proportions is necessary to interfere with male puberty.

Anorexia nervosa is a serious psychiatric disorder characterized by a distorted body image, an obsessive fear of obesity and associated food avoidance. It can cause severe, and sometimes fatal, weight loss. While not restricted by age or gender, anorexia nervosa is more common in girls than boys and most often begins during adolescence. Associated with delayed puberty, it can be accompanied by primary or secondary amenorrhea, depending on the age at onset. The hypogonadotropic hypogonadism of anorexia nervosa is related only in part to the weight loss associated with the disorder. In fact, in postpubertal girls, secondary amenorrhea may precede severe weight loss. Affected individuals will have a reversion of LH secretion to a prepubertal circadian rhythm. Recovery of normal weight will correct many of the coexisting endocrine and metabolic abnormalities, including: low cortisol and triiodothyronine, increased GH and decreased IGF-1 and a blunted pituitary response to trophic hormones. Amenorrhea accompanying anorexia nervosa may persist long after otherwise adequate weight gain. Bulimia nervosa, a variant of anorexia nervosa associated with food gorging, induced vomiting and laxative abuse, produces amenorrhea unassociated with weight loss. This suggests the amenorrhea of anorexia and bulimia nervosa may have a primary hypothalamic origin.

Intense exercise and athletic training may delay or arrest puberty due to inhibition of GnRH secretion. Again, this is more common in girls than boys. Distance runners, gymnasts and dancers are at highest

The Reproductive System at a Glance, Fourth Edition. Linda J. Heffner and Danny J. Schust.

risk. Interruption of training by injury advances puberty before weight gain occurs, suggesting a direct effect of the physical activity on GnRH secretion. Female athletes with normal body weight, but less body fat than nonathletic girls (e.g., swimmers and ice skaters) are also at risk for hypogonadotropic hypogonadism and delayed puberty.

Hypergonadotropic hypogonadism

Gonadal dysgenesis is the most common cause of hypergonadotropic hypogonadism. Primary gonadal failure results in decreased or absent gonadal steroid secretion. Lack of adequate circulating estrogen or androgen reduces negative feedback actions of the hypothalamus on pituitary gland resulting in elevated FSH and LH secretion.

Klinefelter syndrome is the most common cause of gonadal dysgenesis, occurring in 1 in 500–1000 of all phenotypic boys. Typical features of the Klinefelter phenotype are a eunuch-like body habitus, gynecomastia and small testes. The testes of most patients with Klinefelter syndrome have a distinctly limited capacity to secrete testosterone. The Leydig cells in the testis do not respond normally to LH or FSH stimulation; plasma testosterone levels range from 10% of normal in severely eunuchoid boys to about 50% of normal in those less severely affected. Estrogen production is also proportionally elevated compared to the amount of testosterone produced, and gynecomastia is a frequent clinical finding. Boys with Klinefelter syndrome who have circulating testosterone levels in the low normal range will demonstrate puberty and normal height. Those with extremely low circulating testosterone levels will be very tall because of the failure of the epiphyses to close in a timely fashion. Most men with Klinefelter syndrome have normal adrenal androgen production; most will have pubic hair, regardless of circulating testosterone levels.

Boys with Klinefelter syndrome have a progressive loss of spermatogenic activity in the testes after puberty. In normal pubertal boys, about 80% of the seminiferous tubules will contain spermatogonia. In boys with Klinefelter syndrome, only 20% of tubules will contain germ cells. This percentage declines as the tubules gradually sclerose. Adults with Klinefelter syndrome are infertile. Most will require androgen replacement therapy to obtain or maintain an adult male phenotype.

Ninety per cent of men with Klinefelter syndrome have a **47XXY karyotype**. The other 10% display an array of extra X chromosome states. Some have a 46XX karyotype with translocation of the male sex-determining region (SRY) on to the X chromosome (Chapter 5). Still others carry additional X chromosomal material as a mosaicism. Klinefelter mosaics account for the largest proportion of affected men who retain partial testicular function. Fertile 46XY mosaics have been reported.

Turner syndrome is the second most common form of gonadal dysgenesis, occurring in about 1 in 5000 liveborn girls. Typical features of the Turner phenotype include short stature, short webbed neck, micrognathia, broad shield-like chest, anomalies of the left side of the heart (coarctation of the aorta, aortic stenosis, bicuspid aortic valve and dissecting aortic aneurysms) and renal and gastrointestinal anomalies. The ovaries of women with Turner syndrome are typically replaced by connective tissue and are called streak gonads. True streak gonads contain no germ cells and cannot produce reproductive steroids. The uterus and fallopian tubes are present in women with Turner syndrome, but they are typically infantile due to lack of estrogen stimulation. External genitalia and gender orientation are female.

The karyotype of a woman with Turner syndrome is typically **45X**. Like Klinefelter syndrome, structural abnormalities of the X chromosome and mosaicism are also common. Mosaicism and structural abnormalities account for the varied phenotypes reported with the syndrome, which range from that described here to both healthy males and females. Of conceptuses with the 45X karyotype, 99% miscarry. This supports the systemic nature of the abnormalities seen with complete absence of the second sex chromosome and suggests that most surviving Turner syndrome women are undiagnosed mosaics.

Patients with Turner syndrome are usually smaller than average at birth. They grow normally for the first few years after infancy and then begin to slow. Most fail to demonstrate a pubertal growth spurt. This characteristic growth defect appears to be related to the single copy of a gene on the X chromosome known as *PHOG* or *SHOX*. *PHOG* is a transcription factor expressed in osteoblasts.

Some patients with Turner syndrome will have complex karyotypes with mosaicism involving the Y chromosome. The presence of all or part of the Y chromosome may result in phenotypes with the classic Turner phenotype described but ambiguous genitalia or normal male external genitalia. Such patients may have gonadal structures ranging from a streak gonad to a functioning testis. Individuals with a Y cell line or abnormalities involving the Y chromosome are at an increased risk for neoplastic transformation in their gonads. Gonadectomy should be performed at the time of diagnosis.

Genetic disorders of steroidogenesis can cause delayed puberty. They are a large group of rare disorders that cause hypergonadotropic hypogonadism. Because most of these autosomal recessive disorders also affect adrenal steroid biosynthesis, they are more commonly known as the **congenital adrenal hyperplasia (CAH) syndromes**. The CAH syndromes associated with delayed puberty are listed in Table 29.1. All these enzyme defects occur in the steroidogenic pathway between cholesterol and testosterone.

Table 29.1 Classification of delayed or absent puberty

Constitutional delay in growth and puberty

Hypogonadotropic hypogonadism
CNS disorders
    Congenital malformations
    Destructive lesions
Tumors
Radiation therapy
Kallmann syndrome (isolated gonadotropin deficiency)
Multiple pituitary hormone deficiencies
Miscellaneous disorders
Prader–Willi syndrome
Functional gonadotropin deficiency
    Chronic systemic disease and malnutrition
    Hypothyroidism
    Cushing disease
    Diabetes mellitus
    Hyperprolactinemia
    Anorexia nervosa
    Psychogenic amenorrhea
    Exercise-induced amenorrhea
    Fertile eunuch syndrome

Hypergonadotropic hypogonadism
Gonadal dysgenesis
    Turner syndrome
    Klinefelter syndrome
    XX and XY gonadal dysgenesis
Other forms of primary gonadal failure
Disorders of gonadal steroidogenesis = congenital adrenal hyperplasia (CAH)
    Lipoid CAH
    17α-hydroxylase/17,20-lyase deficiency
    3β-hydroxysteroid dehydrogenase deficiency
    20,22-desmolase deficiency

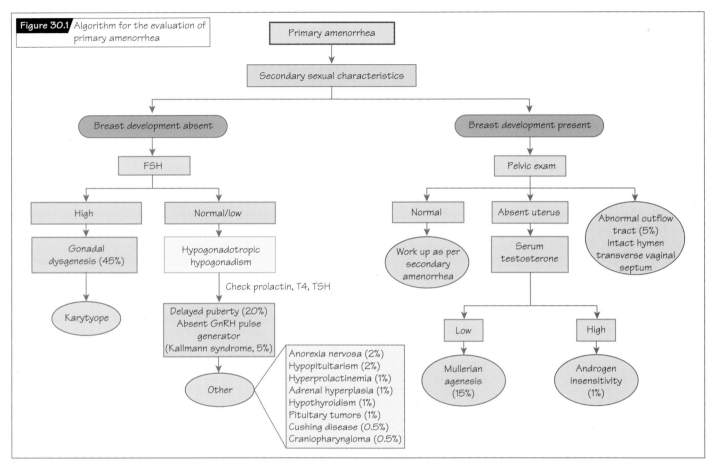

Figure 30.1 Algorithm for the evaluation of primary amenorrhea

Primary amenorrhea is defined as failure to menstruate by age 16 in patients with normal secondary sexual characteristics or the failure to menstruate by age 14 in patients with no signs of sexual maturation (Fig. 30.1). **Secondary amenorrhea** is defined as the absence of three menstrual cycles or the absence of menstrual bleeding for 6 months. The distinction between primary and secondary amenorrhea has traditionally been emphasized because of the higher incidence of genetic and anatomic abnormalities among young women with primary amenorrhea. It remains conceptually useful to make this distinction because of several unique disorders that are found only in patients with one or the other. Still, there is much more overlap in the origins and pathophysiology of the two entities than was originally appreciated. For example, Turner syndrome is a common genetic cause of primary amenorrhea, yet some patients with Turner syndrome have sufficient ovarian reserve to undergo secondary sexual development and menarche before complete ovarian failure results in secondary amenorrhea. Other young women with chronic anovulation due to functional disorders will be classified with primary amenorrhea if the onset of the disorder occurs at puberty. In such cases, it may be more useful to assess the degree to which secondary sexual characteristics have developed in girls with absent menses. Failure of breast and pubic hair development is a sign of delayed or absent puberty and represents a specific subset of reproductive abnormalities (Chapter 29).

As Table 30.1 shows, causes of amenorrhea are extensive and involve all levels of the hypothalamic–pituitary–gonadal–end-organ axis. To avoid confusion, amenorrhea can be divided into two broad categories of abnormalities. The first and largest category is characterized by chronic anovulation. In these patients, a failure to generate cyclic ovarian estrogen and progesterone leads to absent or highly irregular sloughing of an inappropriately stimulated endometrium (Chapters 10 and 14). Chronic anovulation results from four general pathophysiologic mechanisms: (i) the hypothalamus fails to generate a cyclic gonadotropin-releasing hormone (GnRH) signal to the pituitary gland; (ii) the pituitary fails to respond to appropriate signals from the hypothalamus; (iii) the normal sex steroid feedback mechanisms fail to drive the midcycle luteinizing hormone (LH) surge; (iv) interference with gonadal steroid feedback by other endocrine systems. The second, much smaller, category includes end-organ abnormalities that interfere with the ability of these organs to respond to normal cyclic ovarian steroid production and produce visible endometrial bleeding.

Diagnosing the underlying cause of amenorrhea involves sequential determination of the function of each of the potentially affected compartments (uterus and vagina, ovaries, pituitary and hypothalamus). Treatment aims to correct the underlying dysfunction so that menses resume. If it is not possible to establish or restore menstruation, it is very important to assess the hormonal status of untreated or inade-

The Reproductive System at a Glance, Fourth Edition. Linda J. Heffner and Danny J. Schust.

68 © 2014 John Wiley & Sons, Ltd. Published 2014 by John Wiley & Sons, Ltd. Companion Website: www.ataglanceseries.com/reproduction

Table 30.1 Causes of amenorrhea

Hypothalamic disturbances
Primary hypothalamic lesions
   Kallmann syndrome
Secondary hypothalamic lesions
   CNS tumors
Abnormal CNS–hypothalamic interaction
   Anorexia nervosa
   Exercise-induced amenorrhea

Primary pituitary disturbances
Sheehan syndrome (pituitary apoplexy)
Pituitary adenomas
Pituitary tumors
Empty sella syndrome

Secondary pituitary disturbances
Inappropriate gonadal steroid feedback
   Pregnancy
   Contraceptive steroids
   Constant estrogen exposure
   Estrogen excess
   Estrogen-producing tumors
   Aromatase excess
   Estrogen deficiency
   Gene mutations in estrogen receptor
   Aromatase deficiency
   Androgen excess
   Androgen-producing tumors
   Functional excess (adrenal or ovarian)
Inappropriate feedback from other sources
   Polycystic ovary syndrome (PCOS)
   Cushing syndrome
   Hypothyroidism and hyperthyroidism
   Lactation
   Hyperprolactinemia
   Growth hormone excess
   Malnutrition

Gonadal abnormalities
Gonadal failure
   Gonadal dysgenesis
   Menopause
   Ovarian ablation or removal
Gene mutation in LH and FSH receptors

End-organ abnormalities
Uterus
   Müllerian agenesis
   Surgical removal of the uterus
   Endometrial ablation
   Asherman syndrome
Vagina
   Imperforate hymen
   Vaginal septum
Other
   Complete androgen insensitivity (testicular feminization)

quately treated individuals. Chronically hypestrogenic women are at increased risk for osteoporosis (Chapter 24) and women with chronic unopposed estrogen stimulation of their endometrium are at risk for endometrial cancer (Chapter 43). Hormonal therapy to avoid these consequences must be considered in all amenorrheic women.

Etiologies of primary amenorrhea

These are best understood if categorized by: (i) the presence or absence of breast development; (ii) the presence or absence of the cervix and uterus; and (iii) circulating follicle-stimulating hormone (FSH) levels. Figure 30.1 presents an algorithm for evaluating the girl or woman with primary amenorrhea. Unsurprisingly, abnormalities in each of the four compartments mentioned above can be associated with primary amenorrhea.

In order of descending frequency, the most common causes of primary amenorrhea are gonadal dysgenesis, physiologic delay of puberty, Müllerian agenesis, transverse vaginal septum or imperforate hymen, Kallmann syndrome, anorexia nervosa and hypopituitarism. Complete androgen insensitivity, while much rarer than Müllerian agenesis, must be considered in any young woman who has breasts but no uterus. All girls or women with primary amenorrhea and an elevated FSH must have a karyotype performed to determine whether 2X chromosomes are present or if a Y chromosome (or even a piece of a Y chromosome) is present. The presence of any Y chromosome genes and an intraabdominal gonad, regardless of its phenotype, confers a risk for germ-cell tumor development. These gonads must be surgically removed, typically at the time of diagnosis.

Gonadal dysgenesis with a pure 45X karyotype can usually be diagnosed because of the other physical features of Turner syndrome (Chapters 27 and 29). Other abnormalities of the sex chromosomes can also cause amenorrhea, including 45X/46XX, other mosaics, and 46XY with a missing SRY locus (Chapter 5). **Müllerian agenesis**, also known as the Mayer–Rokitansky–Kuster–Hauser syndrome, is characterized by a complete absence of the female internal genitalia, including the vagina, uterus and fallopian tubes, in a chromosomally normal female. Its biologic cause is unknown. **Transverse vaginal septa** are thought to result from failure of the vaginal plate to resorb at the site where the Müllerian ducts fuse with it to form the cervix (Chapters 6 and 27). **Kallmann syndrome** is a developmental abnormality of the central nervous system (CNS) in which those neurosecretory cells destined to become the GnRH pulse generator fail to migrate from their origins in the olfactory placode to the median basal hypothalamus (Chapter 29). In addition to reproductive abnormalities, individuals with Kallmann syndrome also cannot smell because of the inadequate development or complete absence of the olfactory neurons that develop from the same anlagen. **Anorexia nervosa** or extreme exercise and their consequent hypothalamic suppression can cause delayed or absent puberty if the disorder begins in childhood, primary amenorrhea if it begins during puberty, or secondary amenorrhea if it begins later in adolescence. **Hypopituitarism** most commonly results from CNS tumors and can present as either absent or delayed puberty or amenorrhea depending on timing of onset and the rate of tumor growth. **Complete androgen insensitivity (AI)**, previously called **testicular feminization**, is a rare X-linked disorder caused by mutations in the androgen receptor that make it unresponsive to androgen. Although they can make testosterone and other androgens, patients with complete AI cannot exhibit androgen activity at central or peripheral target tissues. Genitalia fail to masculinize during embryogenesis and androgens cannot exert negative feedback on FSH production by the pituitary gland. Individuals with complete AI are phenotypic girls and will develop breasts at puberty because the androgens secreted by their overstimulated testes can be converted peripherally to estrogens. They do not have a uterus. Therefore, they will not menstruate and will present with primary amenorrhea in the presence of adequate breast development.

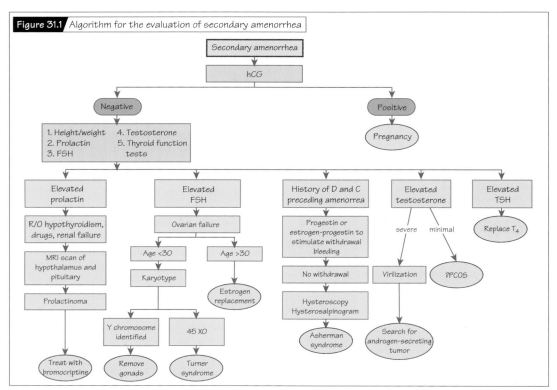

Figure 31.1 Algorithm for the evaluation of secondary amenorrhea

The etiologies of primary and secondary amenorrhea often overlap. Those more commonly associated with primary amenorrhea are discussed in Chapter 30. Most secondary amenorrhea results from anovulation. The most common reason is **pregnancy**; this etiology should be evaluated before considering any other cause. An algorithm for evaluating secondary amenorrhea is shown in Fig. 31.1.

Polycystic ovary syndrome (PCOS) is the most common cause of chronic anovulatory amenorrhea. It is a disorder characterized by amenorrhea or oligomenorrhea, physical signs of hyperandrogenism (hirsutism, acne) and the presence of enlarged polycystic ovaries. PCOS pathophysiology can be linked to the combination of: (i) exaggerated pulsatile gonadotropin-releasing hormone (GnRH) secretion, causing elevated circulating luteinizing hormone (LH) and an increased LH:FSH (follicle-stimulating hormone) ratio; and (ii) defects in insulin signaling for glucose transport and lipolysis, causing insulin resistance (Fig. 31.2).

The mechanism for the exaggerated GnRH pulse frequency and amplitude is unknown, but its appearance at puberty suggests an intrinsic, primary pathogenic defect. Pituitary gonadotrophs are exquisitely sensitive to the frequency and amplitude of GnRH pulses and the pattern present in patients with PCOS causes a relative increase in the secretion of LH with respect to FSH. Ovarian theca cells respond to LH by increasing cholesterol conversion to androgens (Chapter 2). Conversion of these androgens to estrogen in the ovary is reduced by a decrease in aromatase activity that accompanies the relative FSH deficiency. Hyperandrogenism, in turn, causes local follicular arrest and anovulation and systemic stimulation of sex steroid-responsive hair follicles, resulting in hirsutism and acne. The androgen-producing theca cells in the ovaries of patients with PCOS become hyperplastic and are surrounded by an increased number of developmentally arrested primary and secondary follicles, which can be documented ultrasonographically as enlarged ovaries encircled by a "string of pearls."

Insulin abnormalities are as important in PCOS as are those in the GnRH pulse generator. In fact, therapy with insulin sensitizers can correct both metabolic and hormonal alterations. In untreated patients, cellular defects in glucose transport result in transient hyperglycemia and reactive hyperinsulinemia. Insulin synergizes with LH to stimulate androgen production by theca cells and inhibits the hepatic production of sex hormone-binding globulin (SHBG), thereby increasing circulating free androgen. The cellular lipolytic defect in women with PCOS results from a reduction in β-adrenoceptor density on adipocytes and causes increased fat storage and obesity. Obesity, present in over half of women with PCOS, amplifies the abnormalities of insulin resistance and hyperinsulinemia.

The somatotropic (growth) axis has also been implicated in PCOS pathogenesis. Growth hormone (GH) and its peripheral mediators, insulin-like growth factors (IGFs), their binding proteins (IGFBPs) and their receptors enhance steroidogenesis by ovarian theca and granulosa cells. Nonobese patients with PCOS have exaggerated GH pulse amplitudes, similar to their exaggerated GnRH pulses. In contrast, obese women with PCOS have hyperinsulinemia but blunted GH secretion. Because insulin interacts with the IGF system at multiple levels and can bind to the IGF-1 receptor, hyperinsulinemia mimics GH excess. In either case, there will be increased somatotropic activity and excessive androgen production in the ovary.

At least 50% of women with PCOS also show functional adrenal hyperandrogenism, making differentiation of PCOS from late-onset congenital adrenal hyperplasia (CAH) difficult. The exact nature of the adrenal dysfunction in PCOS is unclear, but evidence points to an

The Reproductive System at a Glance, Fourth Edition. Linda J. Heffner and Danny J. Schust.

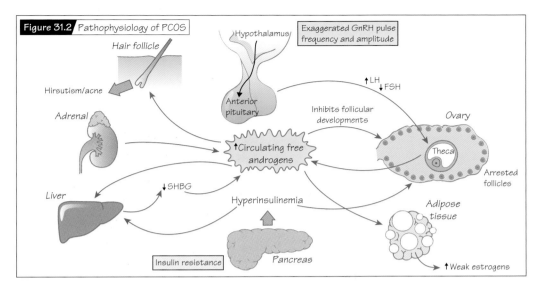

Figure 31.2 Pathophysiology of PCOS

Hair follicle

Hirsutism/acne

Adrenal

Liver

Hypothalamus

Exaggerated GnRH pulse frequency and amplitude

Anterior pituitary

↑LH ↓FSH

↑Circulating free androgens

↓SHBG

Inhibits follicular developments

Ovary

Theca

Arrested follicles

Hyperinsulinemia

Insulin resistance

Pancreas

Adipose tissue

↑Weak estrogens

increase in P450c17 activities in the zona reticularis of the adrenal cortex. LH, insulin and IGF-1 stimulate this enzyme in the ovary to produce androgens. Patients with PCOS with functional adrenal hyperandrogenism have exaggerated adrenal androgen production in response to adrenocorticotropic hormone (ACTH) stimulation. Excessive adrenal androgen production during adrenarche may trigger the onset of PCOS in these women by increasing serum androstenedione that is converted extragonadally to the weak estrogen estrone. Inappropriate estrone production, in turn, may produce a premature and pathologic trophic effect on the reproductive axis, causing PCOS at puberty.

Treatment of PCOS aims to reduce insulin resistance, to establish ovulation when fertility is desired, and to prevent prolonged unopposed estrogen activity during anovulation and its associated risk for endometrial hyperplasia and cancer. Antiandrogens may be required to treat acne and hirsutism caused by hyperandrogenism.

All **functional hypothalamic disorders** are associated with decreased GnRH pulse frequency and amplitude. CNS input to the GnRH pulse generator can be disrupted by the psychogenic starvation of anorexia nervosa, by strenuous exercise and by stress. Infiltrative diseases of the hypothalamus such as lymphoma and histiocytosis, while rare, can also disrupt GnRH secretion.

Amenorrhea resulting from **excessive prolactin secretion** can arise from multiple abnormalities, including prolactin secreting microadenomas and macroadenomas, hypothyroidism and use of a wide variety of medications (Chapter 32).

Premature ovarian failure (POF), the cessation of menses before age 40 in the absence of genetic abnormalities, accounts for 10% of the cases of secondary amenorrhea. Women with POF typically exhibit amenorrhea, elevated gonadotropin levels and decreased circulating estrogens. Many will have hot flashes. In most cases, the exact cause for ovarian failure will not be found. Some cases of POF are associated with autoimmune diseases such as Hashimoto thyroiditis, Addison disease, hypoparathyroidism and myasthenia gravis, or may be part of a polyendocrine syndrome. Antibodies to gonadotropins and gonadotropin receptors have been found in some patients. Others lack antibodies, but carry genetic mutations in LH or FSH receptors. Occasionally, ovarian failure is temporary and pregnancies have followed an apparent cessation of ovarian function.

Intrauterine synechiae or adhesions occlude the uterine cavity in **Asherman syndrome**. Because the condition may develop after an intrauterine infection or postpartum curettage for heavy bleeding, it is thought that these procedures can inappropriately remove deep endometrial layers and destroy the basal crypts and glands necessary for endometrial regeneration. The scarring associated with Asherman syndrome can totally obliterate the uterine cavity, although milder degrees of scarring can also cause amenorrhea. Direct injury and local paracrine dysfunction may both be involved.

Hypothyroidism is associated with menstrual irregularities and amenorrhea. Thyroxine can increase estrogen and progesterone secretion by cultured human granulosa cells and thyroid hormone deficiency may adversely alter ovarian steroidogenesis. Also, the increased hypothalamic secretion of thyrotropin-releasing factor (TRF) accompanying primary hypothyroidism will stimulate prolactin secretion. The resulting hyperprolactinemia inhibits pulsatile GnRH secretion and causes menstrual irregularities (Chapter 32).

CAH, Cushing syndrome and **obesity** all are associated with excess androgen production. Although adrenal androgens (DHEA and DHEA-S; Chapter 2) are relatively weak, their presence in pathologic amounts can lead to significant androgenic effects. Most effects occur after conversion to more potent androgens and estrogens in peripheral cells such as adipocytes. In women, the resultant noncyclic, gonadotropin-independent sex steroid secretion interferes with normal cyclic secretion of FSH and LH by the pituitary and causes oligo- or anovulation.

In **empty sella syndrome**, the bony structure surrounding the pituitary gland is flattened and appears enlarged and empty. Some patients with an apparently empty sella have headaches and no endocrine dysfunction. Others have single or multiple endocrinopathies including gonadotropin deficiencies and hyperprolactinemia. The cause of empty sella syndrome is unknown.

The pituitary gland is particularly vulnerable to **hypotensive injury during pregnancy**. Pituitary infarction associated with postpartum hemorrhage and shock is called **Sheehan syndrome**. In Sheehan's original description, patients presented with panhypopituitarism. Such severe forms of Sheehan syndrome are rarely encountered in modern obstetric practice, but partial forms occasionally are. The severity of the injury determines the specific pituitary functions affected and loss occurs in a fairly predictable order. Most vulnerable is GH secretion. More severe cases will impair, in decreasing order of frequency, prolactin, thyroid-stimulating hormone and ACTH secretion.

Figure 32.1 (a) Regulators of prolactin secretion

Figure 32.1 (b) An MRI image of the brain showing a pituitary macroadenoma

Hyperprolactinemia is a common clinical problem. Cases resulting from inappropriate prolactin secretion by the pituitary gland are the third most frequently diagnosed cause of chronic anovulation and secondary amenorrhea. There are many etiologies for this condition; some result from serious underlying pathology and others from reversible functional disorders.

Control of prolactin secretion is dominated by tonic inhibition and there is no regulation by classic negative feedback from its target organs. These characteristics are unique among pituitary hormones. The major inhibitor of prolactin secretion is dopamine and the two major stimuli are estrogen and thyrotropin-releasing hormone (TRH). Numerous other neurohormonal regulators must also be considered when elucidating the mechanisms by which hyperprolactinemia develops.

Regulation of prolactin secretion

Embryonic differentiation of the lactotroph is under the control of the pituitary-specific transcriptional factor Pit-1. While Pit-1 regulates prolactin gene transcription by binding directly to the prolactin promoter, other regulators of prolactin gene expression use alternative pathways (Fig. 32.1a). Dopamine released into the pituitary portal system binds to a G_1-protein-coupled receptor and inhibits adenylate cyclase and phospholipase C. Acting as a neurohormone, rather than a neurotransmitter, dopamine reduces prolactin synthesis and prolactin release by the pituitary lactotrope. TRH acts through a second lactotroph cell membrane receptor to activate phospholipase C. In contrast to dopamine, TRH increases prolactin gene transcription and release of prolactin hormone from its storage granules. The effect of TRH is modulated by thyroid hormone such that decreases in T_3 and T_4 enhance prolactin release and increased concentrations of T_3 and T_4 decrease prolactin secretion. Estradiol acts through a third mechanism, binding not to a membrane receptor but to a nuclear receptor.

The hormone receptor complex then interacts with estrogen response elements upstream of the prolactin gene. Estradiol also interferes with dopaminergic activation of its receptor and increases the concentration of TRH receptors on lactotrophs. Both actions potentiate the stimulatory effects of the sex steroid.

Like dopamine, γ-aminobutyric acid (GABA) and glucocorticoids inhibit prolactin secretion. The mechanism by which GABA acts as a prolactin inhibitory factor is unknown. Like estrogen, glucocorticoids act through nuclear receptors to inhibit prolactin gene transcription. Vasoactive peptide (VIP), oxytocin, angiotensin II (AgII) and serotonin all increase prolactin secretion. VIP employs two mechanisms: it stimulates oxytocin release via the hypothalamus and it interferes with dopamine inhibition of adenylate cyclase. AgII acts on a specific membrane receptor on the lactotroph to provoke rapid release of presynthesized prolactin. It is a more potent secretagogue for prolactin than TRH. Serotonin released by the dorsal raphe nucleus also stimulates prolactin release but not its synthesis. Here, serotonin activity occurs independent of dopamine pathways.

In the physiologic state, fine tuning of prolactin secretion is determined by the balance between the prolactin inhibitory factors (PIF) and the prolactin-releasing factors (PRF). Any disorder that alters the balanced secretion of these regulatory compounds will result in altered prolactin secretion. Regardless of its cause, hyperprolactinemia can interfere with hypothalamic–pituitary function and result in hypogonadism with or without galactorrhea. The fact that women with prolactin-induced amenorrhea are hypo-estrogenic but do not experience hot flashes suggests that one mechanism by which prolactin alters hypothalamic–pituitary function is via modulation of central neurotransmission. The hypothalamic dopaminergic and opioid systems that regulate gonadotropin-releasing hormone (GnRH) pulsatility are likely to be involved in this effect.

The Reproductive System at a Glance, Fourth Edition. Linda J. Heffner and Danny J. Schust.

Table 32.1 Conditions associated with increased prolactin secretion

Physiologic causes	Pharmacologic causes		Pathologic causes	
Sleep	Estrogen therapy	CNS dopamine depleting	Hypothalamic lesions	Pituitary tumors
Feeding	Anesthesia	agents	Craniopharyngioma	Cushing disease
Exercise	Dopamine receptor blockers	Methyldopa	Glioma	Acromegaly
Stress	Domperidone	Monoamine oxidase	Granulomas	Prolactinoma
Coitus	Risperidone	inhibitors	Histiocytosis	Nonsecreting adenomas
Menstrual cycle	Haloperidol	Reserpine	Sarcoid	Neural reflexes
Pregnancy	Metoclopramide	Opiates (codeine,	Tuberculosis	Chest wall injury
Postpartum	Phenothiazines	morphine)	Pituitary stalk transection	Herpes zoster neuritis
Nursing	Pimozide	Stimulators of serotonergic	Head injury or	Upper abdominal
Fetal/neonatal	Sulpride	system	postsurgical	surgery
	Amisulpride	Amphetamines	Irradiation damage	Hypothyroidism
	Select calcium channel	Hallucinogens	Pseudocyesis	Renal failure
	blockers	Histamine H_2 receptor		Ectopic production
	Verapamil	antagonists		Bronchogenic
		Cimetidine		carcinoma
		Ranitidine		Hypernephroma
		Nizatidine		
		Famotidine		

Physiologic hyperprolactinemia

Most physiologic hyperprolactinemia is transient and of no clinical consequence. High physiologic concentrations of plasma prolactin occur at night and result from both an intrinsic circadian rhythm and sleep-entrained prolactin release. High protein meals at midday, but not in the morning, induce prolactin release through an unknown mechanism. Physical and emotional stress, including exercise, hypoglycemia and anesthesia are associated with elevations in prolactin secretion. Orgasm promotes prolactin secretion, but only in women. Pregnancy is associated with a marked elevation of prolactin secretion that persists into the immediate postpartum period (Chapter 23). Of all the physiologic hyperprolactinemic states, only lactation is associated with amenorrhea.

Pharmacologic hyperprolactinemia

Medications that interfere with dopaminergic inhibition of the pituitary lactotroph can cause hyperprolactinemia. Any drug that decreases the synthesis of dopamine, enhances its metabolism, increases its reuptake or interferes with its binding to its receptor will reduce the action of dopamine. When the inhibitory activity of dopamine on the pituitary lactotroph is blocked, prolactin secretion increases. All of the medications listed in Table 32.1 can inhibit dopamine action and cause hyperprolactinemia. Clinical manifestations of pharmacologic hyperprolactinemia include galactorrhea and menstrual irregularities. Menstrual dysfunction may be severe enough to result in amenorrhea.

Pathologic hyperprolactinemia

Lesions in the hypothalamus or in the pituitary gland can cause hyperprolactinemia. Those in the hypothalamus typically do so by interfering with dopamine delivery to the pituitary gland. Tumors are the most frequent of the pituitary causes of hyperprolactinemia; the prolactin-secreting adenoma is the most common of these (Fig. 32.1b). Prolactin-secreting adenomas (prolactinomas) are classified by size: microadenomas are less than 1 cm in size and macroadenomas are greater than 1 cm. These tumors can occur in both men and women, but are more common in women. In women they cause galactorrhea, amenorrhea, headache and visual field defects. In men they cause headache, visual field changes and impotence. They are often larger at diagnosis in men than in women because symptom onset is typically late in men. Prolactinomas are usually benign. Pituitary adenomas that

produce adrenocorticotropic hormone (Cushing disease) and growth hormone (acromegaly) may also cause hyperprolactinemia.

Primary hypothyroidism can also cause hyperprolactinemia. The decrease in circulating thyroid hormone that accompanies thyroid gland dysfunction diminishes negative feedback on the hypothalamus and pituitary gland. This results in an increase in TRH and thyroid-stimulating hormone secretion. Excessive TRH can override the normal dopamine-dominated inhibition of prolactin secretion through direct, receptor-mediated effects on the pituitary lactotroph. A significant proportion of patients with chronic renal failure will have hyperprolactinemia. While the etiology of this effect remains incompletely described, patients with chronic renal failure appear to have circulating serum factors that interfere with dopaminergic inhibition of prolactin synthesis and secretion.

Treatment of hyperprolactinemia is directed toward correction of the underlying cause. A notable exception to this rule involves the management of the prolactin-secreting pituitary adenoma. Resection of these tumors is associated with a high frequency of recurrence of the hyperprolactinemia. Medical management is typically safer and more effective and involves use of oral dopamine agonists (e.g., bromocriptine, cabergoline). It is important to remember that men and women with hyperprolactinemia are hypogonadal due to the associated abnormalities in the hypothalamic–pituitary–gonadal axis. This hypogonadal state places them at significant risk for osteoporosis (Chapter 24) and requires continuation of therapy for as long as the hyperprolactinemia persists.

Galactorrhea

Galactorrhea describes the secretion of breast milk in states unassociated with nursing. Galactorrhea can result from hyperprolactinemia or from excessive sensitivity of the breast to normal circulating levels of prolactin. If galactorrhea is associated with amenorrhea, then hyperprolactinemia is likely the cause. If galactorrhea occurs in the presence of normal ovulatory cycles, then excessive sensitivity of the breast to normal circulating amounts of prolactin is more likely. The three most common causes of hyperprolactinemia resulting in galactorrhea are: (i) a pituitary adenoma, (ii) medications interfering with dopamine action and (iii) hypothyroidism. Galactorrhea can be suppressed by the use of dopamine agonists.

Figure 33.1 Dual control elements of human sexual motivation

Prior to 1980, sexual dysfunction of any cause was lumped under the term "impotence" for men and "frigidity" for women. Since then, the classification of sexual disorders has evolved and is now based on the physiologically oriented, four-phase model of human sexuality (Chapter 15). This classification divides the sexual dysfunction syndromes into disorders of desire, disorders of excitement/arousal and disorders of orgasm. The fourth phase of the human sexual response, resolution, is rarely disturbed. Sexual desire disorders include hyperactive and hypoactive sexual drive (libido) and sexual aversion. Excitement phase disorders include erectile dysfunction, dyspareunia and vaginismus. Orgasmic disorders include inhibited orgasm in women and premature ejaculation in men.

Sexual desire disorders

Normal sexual drive can be thought of as a balance between an "erotic motor," which incites a desire for sexual activity, and a "sexual brake," which keeps urges in check. These excitatory and inhibitory signals appear to converge upon specific centers in the hypothalamus and limbic system to produce a continuum of sexual desire. It is probably only the polar ends of this range that are abnormal (Fig. 33.1). There is no specific test for abnormal sexual desire. Instead, the diagnosis of a sexual desire disorder is based on the subjective reporting of abnormal libido that results in individual distress or interpersonal difficulty.

The two formally recognized sexual desire disorders are hypoactive sexual desire disorder (HSDD) and sexual aversion disorder. HSDD is defined as persistently or recurrently deficient (or absent) sexual fantasies or desire for sexual activity. Sexual aversion disorder is the persistent or recurrent extreme aversion to, and avoidance of, all (or almost all) genital sexual contact with a sexual partner. Of patients seeking treatment for sexual desire disorders, 79% have HSDD, 20% have sexual aversion disorder and 1% have hyperactive sexual desires. The causes of sexual desire disorders may be either organic or psychosocial. Organic causes include testosterone deficiency, chronic illness, certain centrally acting medications and underlying psychiatric disturbances. Psychogenic causes involve psychologically repressive stimuli such as anxiety, anger, perception of a partner as repulsive, or previous negative sexual experiences.

Treatment of the sexual desire disorders is directed first toward evaluation and correction of any underlying organic problem. Psychotherapy may be useful in the treatment of sexual desire disorders of nonorganic etiologies. Patients with long-standing sexual dysfunction of organic etiology often develop concomitant psychosocial issues. Individual or group counseling may be extremely useful as adjunctive therapy in these patients.

Erectile dysfunction (impotence)

Erectile dysfunction (ED) is the recurrent inability of a man to get and keep an erection sufficient for intercourse. ED is mild if a man can usually get and keep an erection, moderate if he can only can get or keep an erection sometimes and complete if he never can. Risk factors for ED include aging, chronic illnesses, a variety of medications and cigarette smoking. It is a common problem among older men; estimates report that 50% of 40- to 70-year-old men have some degree of ED. Even more are affected after the age of 70.

ED can occur because of vasculogenic, neurogenic, hormonal or psychogenic problems. Eighty per cent of the diagnosable conditions leading to ED are organic. They include, in decreasing order of frequency, atherosclerosis, diabetes, hypertension, medication side

The Reproductive System at a Glance, Fourth Edition. Linda J. Heffner and Danny J. Schust.

74 © 2014 John Wiley & Sons, Ltd. Published 2014 by John Wiley & Sons, Ltd. Companion Website: www.ataglanceseries.com/reproduction

effects, prostate surgery, hyperthyroidism and hypothyroidism, hyperprolactinemia and hypogonadism. While depression is present in 60% of men with ED, it is often unclear whether this mood disorder is the cause or the result of long-standing ED.

Successful penile erection involves the activity of autonomic nerves upon the vascular smooth muscle of the penis. Relaxation of penile vascular smooth muscle allows blood to flow into the penis. Here it remains trapped and erection occurs (Chapter 13). Most of the organic causes of ED involve neuropathies of the autonomic nervous system, vascular compromise or, occasionally, testosterone deficiency. Psychogenic ED involves abnormal central inhibition of the erectile mechanism in the absence of demonstrable physical abnormality. The presence of morning erections in a man with ED may suggest a psychogenic etiology. Drugs that produce ED are myriad and typically affect the neural reflex pathways necessary for integrating the erection. Examples of medications associated with ED include antidepressants, antipsychotics, sedatives, antianxiety medications, antihypertensives and anticonvulsants. Alcohol and street drugs, including amphetamines, cocaine, marijuana, methadone and heroin, can also cause ED.

Until recently, treatment options for ED were limited to medication changes, implantable erection devices, intracavernosal injections of prostaglandins and psychotherapy. The discovery that the drug sildenafil can facilitate and maintain erections in impotent men has changed the treatment of ED dramatically. Sildenafil was originally tried as an antiangina medication and found to be ineffective. The study subjects were reluctant to turn in their leftover pills and soon the drug's unexpected side effect was uncovered. Since then sildenafil, and related drugs, have been shown to be effective in the treatment of ED and have become widely available for this use. These medications work by inhibiting phosphodiesterase type V (PDE5), a cyclic guanosine monophosphate (cGMP) metabolizing enzyme found predominantly in the penis. Nitric oxide (NO) activates guanylate cyclase in the penis, increasing cGMP, the major mediator of the vascular relaxation necessary for penile erection. The longer cGMP stays around, the longer the duration of erection. Blockade of cGMP metabolism promotes and maintains NO proerectile activity. PDE5 inhibitors will not cause erections in the absence of sexual stimuli.

Premature ejaculation

This is a disorder characterized by ejaculation that occurs with minimal sexual stimulation after penetration and before the man wishes it. This must occur on multiple occasions over time to warrant diagnosis. When making the diagnosis, the man's age, the novelty of the sexual partner and circumstances and his frequency of sexual activity must be taken into account. Premature ejaculation is reported by 10–35% of men seeking help for sexual dysfunction. Unlike ED, which increases with age, premature ejaculation decreases with age.

The exact cause of premature ejaculation is unknown. The only demonstrable physiologic correlate of premature ejaculation is that men reporting this disorder ejaculate at a lower level of sexual arousal than do control men.

Retrograde ejaculation

In men with retrograde ejaculation, semen travels backwards into the bladder rather than out of the penile shaft during ejaculation because the bladder neck does not close appropriately during or after emission. The most common cause of retrograde ejaculation is inability of the bladder neck to close following transurethral prostatectomy (TURP). Damage to penile innervation during prostate surgery, diabetic neu-

ropathy and the use of anticholinergic medications are neurologic causes of the condition. Retrograde ejaculation does not require intervention unless fertility is desired (Chapter 34).

Dyspareunia

Patients with dyspareunia experience recurrent or persistent genital pain before, during (the most common) or after sexual intercourse. Of women seeking help with sexual problems, 10–30% report dyspareunia, while only 1% of men report the problem. Because dyspareunia is reported far more frequently in women than in men, much more is known about its etiologies and interventional approaches in women.

Dyspareunia may reflect a physical or psychogenic problem. Details of whether the symptoms are lifelong or acquired, generalized or situational are helpful in identifying the potential etiology. Organic causes of dyspareunia include the presence of hymeneal remnants, pelvic tumors, endometriosis, pelvic inflammatory disease and vulvar vestibulitis. Hypoestrogenic states associated with menopause, the early postpartum period, use of very low dose oral contraceptives and prior treatment with chemotherapy may also cause dyspareunia. Psychosocial problems that result in dyspareunia may include poor self-esteem and body image, guilt and prior sexual abuse or trauma. Interpersonal factors between the couple, including anger, distrust and poor communication, may also be responsible.

Treatment of dyspareunia is directed toward evaluation and correction of underlying organic problems. Psychotherapy may be useful in the treatment of dyspareunia of nonorganic causes. It may also be useful as concomitant therapy for those with primary organic causes.

Vaginismus

Women with vaginismus experience recurrent involuntary spasms of the pelvic muscles of the outer third of the vaginal barrel of such severity that intercourse is painful or impossible. Typically, these occur in anticipation of intercourse or during penetration. In some women with severe vaginismus, spasms can also occur during a pelvic examination or tampon insertion.

Vaginismus occurs in 0.5–5% of women. There are significant intercultural differences. Lifelong vaginismus is a rare clinical entity in North America and most of Western Europe. It is relatively common in Ireland, Eastern Europe and Latin America. It is the most commonly reported cause of unconsummated marriages.

Like dyspareunia, vaginismus can have either an organic or psychosocial etiology. The organic bases of the disorder are the same as those of dyspareunia. In fact, most experts believe that vaginismus begins as dyspareunia and escalates to vaginismus through a classic conditioning process. In this view, a woman first has pain on intercourse (unconditioned stimulus) and this leads to a natural self-protecting tightening of the vaginal muscles (conditioned response). Over time, stimuli associated with vaginal penetration can become conditioned stimuli and provoke the conditioned reflex muscle spasms. In severe cases, conditioned stimuli can even include thoughts of sexual intercourse.

Not all cases of vaginismus are classically conditioned from an organic cause. Many psychosocial contributors have been suggested, including guilt, religious constraints, responses to a partner's sexual dysfunction, prior sexual trauma, concerns about sexual orientation and fears of pregnancy, sexually transmitted diseases and trauma.

Like dyspareunia, treatment of vaginismus is directed toward evaluation and correction of any underlying organic problem, and psychotherapy.

34 Infertility

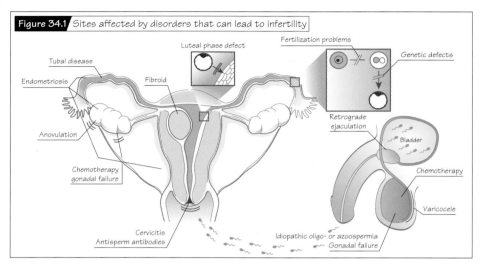

Figure 34.1 Sites affected by disorders that can lead to infertility

Infertility is defined as a diminished capacity to conceive and bear a child. It is not equivalent to sterility, the absolute and irreversible inability to conceive. Clinically, a couple is considered infertile if they are unable to conceive after 12 months of unprotected, frequent coitus.

Many factors contribute to infertility (Fig. 34.1). Diseases that affect only females account for about half of infertile couples and diseases that only affect males about one-third. About 10% of couples will have disorders in both the male and the female partner. Some 10–15% of couples have no identifiable cause for their infertility or will become pregnant during the evaluation. Specific disorders causing infertility include those involving each of the major physiologic events necessary to produce a pregnancy: (i) production of a healthy egg; (ii) production of healthy sperm; (iii) transportation of the sperm to the site of fertilization; (iv) transportation of the zygote to the uterus for implantation; (v) successful implantation in a receptive endometrium; (v) presence of other conditions, some immunologic, that can interfere with one or more of the other events.

Oocyte abnormalities

The main cause of female infertility due to oocyte abnormalities is a failure to ovulate regularly or, in some cases, at all. Those disorders that result in oligo-ovulation or anovulation are also causes of amenorrhea (see Chapters 30 and 31), and fall into three categories: hypothalamic dysfunction, pituitary disease and ovarian dysfunction.

Common hypothalamic causes of anovulation include abnormalities of weight and body composition, strenuous exercise, stress and travel. Pituitary or endocrine disorders associated with anovulation are hyperprolactinemia and hypothyroidism. The two most common known causes of ovarian dysfunction are polycystic ovary syndrome and premature ovarian failure. Oocyte abnormalities more complex than simple anovulation cause the fairly rapid decline in fertility that occurs as women enter their 40s.

Female anatomic abnormalities

Fallopian tubal disease is usually the result of inflammatory scarring of the fallopian tubes. This may be caused by pelvic inflammatory disease, appendicitis with rupture, septic abortion, previous surgery

and, occasionally, previous use of an intrauterine device. The most common site of tubal blockage is the distal fimbriated end of the tube. These blockages are typically associated with additional pelvic adhesions and may affect up to 20% of the women in infertile couples. Purposeful, surgically-induced blockage occurs with surgical sterilization; some women regret their contraceptive decision post-tubal sterilization and present to the fertility specialist requesting reversal.

Endometriosis is a common disorder, characterized by the presence of tissue resembling endometrium outside of its normal position lining the uterus. The glands and stroma of endometriosis are usually responsive to gonadal hormones and the biochemical changes the steroids induce in this ectopic endometrium mimic those seen in endometrium within the uterine cavity. Increased prostaglandin production by perimenstrual and menstrual endometriotic lesions is thought to promote the inflammation, fibrosis and adhesion formation characteristic of the disorder. Endometriosis lesions can be found almost anywhere in the pelvis but are most common on the peritoneal surfaces covering the pouch of Douglas, bladder, ovaries, fallopian tubes, bowel and appendix. Women with endometriosis can present with pelvic pain, adnexal masses (endometriomas), infertility, or any combination of these.

Uterine **leiomyomas**, also known as fibroids or uterine myomas, are benign smooth muscle tumors of the uterus. They are the most common pelvic tumor in women, and may be located anywhere within the wall of the uterus or may hang from a stalk containing the blood supply to the tumour (pedunculated leiomyomas). Pedunculated leiomyomas may hang from the outside of the uterus or may project into the endometrial cavity. Those leiomyomas that distort the uterine cavity (submucosal in location) or physically obstruct fallopian tubes are most closely associated with decreased fecundity.

Male factors

A **varicocele** is a dilatation of the pampiniform plexus of veins that drain the contents of the scrotum. Varicoceles appear to reduce semen quality in some men and their correction improves semen quality. The ultimate effect of correction on fertility is less clear. Varicoceles may adversely affect semen quality by exposing the testis to temperatures higher than those in nonaffected men or by exposing the testis to

The Reproductive System at a Glance, Fourth Edition. Linda J. Heffner and Danny J. Schust.

abnormally high concentrations of gonadotoxic substances. Both effects appear to result from decreased venous efflux from the affected testis.

Blockage of the vas deferens or epididymis can result from congenital abnormalities (i.e., mutations in the cystic fibrosis transmembrane regulator gene; Chapter 26), from infection-associated scarring, or from inadvertent surgical ligation at the time of inguinal surgery. Purposeful, surgically induced blockage occurs with vasectomy; some vasectomized men regret their contraceptive decision and present to the fertility specialist requesting reversal.

Damage to the bladder neck or injury to the lumbar sympathetic nerves involved in the ejaculation reflex may cause retrograde ejaculation, as may neurologic conditions such as multiple sclerosis if they inhibit normal innervation to the bladder neck. With retrograde ejaculation, sperm pass into the bladder upon ejaculation rather than exiting from the penile urethra. Therapy is unnecessary if fertility is not desired. If it is, medical therapies may augment bladder neck closure. If these fail, sperm may be harvested from alkalinized urine.

Men may also produce very few or no sperm because of inadequate hormonal stimulation of the testis or because of gonadal failure. Men with hypogonadotropic hypogonadism may have pituitary gland or hypothalamic defects (e.g., Kallmann syndrome). They fail to secrete gonadotropins and so lack appropriate testicular function. These men are good candidates for treatment with exogenous gonadotropins. Most will respond and produce viable sperm. Men with gonadal failure (e.g. Klinefelter syndrome; 47XXY; Chapters 26 and 29), have few therapeutic options. Some with oligospermia or azospermia will never discover the cause of their disorder.

Implantation abnormalities

Implantation abnormalities encompass a group of endometrial and embryonic defects that interfere with the complex communication occurring between these entities early in the postconception period. Luteal phase deficiency (LPD) is the most discussed of the endometrial disorders that may directly impact implantation. LPD describes a group of endometrial maturation abnormalities that have been associated with subfertility and recurrent pregnancy loss. In LPD of ovarian etiology, abnormal follicular development and ovulation lead to a relative deficiency in progesterone production. This delays or minimizes the effects of progesterone in converting the endometrium into a secretory organ receptive to implantation. Diagnostic tests for the condition are presently suboptimal.

Other factors

Many other factors can influence fecundity; several of these are immunologic. Antisperm antibodies have been identified in some patients with infertility but have also been detected in fertile couples. Their etiologic role and treatment remain unclear. Inflammatory cells recruited into cervical mucus in response to cervical infections may affect sperm function, perhaps through release of cytokines. Some women develop antibodies against negatively charged phospholipids commonly encountered in cell membranes. These antiphospholipid antibodies can inhibit placental formation, activate the complement cascade and promote thromboses in small vessels leading to local ischemia and infarction. Although antiphospholipid antibodies more typically result in recurrent early miscarriage, some women experience loss so early as not to know they are even pregnant. In these women, the antiphospholipid syndrome may initially manifest itself clinically as infertility.

Genetic abnormalities such as the androgen insensitivity (Chapter 26) and gonadal dysgenesis syndromes (Chapters 26 and 27) can also cause infertility. Gonadotoxin exposure, including exposure to radiation, cigarette smoke and chemotherapeutic agents, can cause gonadal dysfunction and impaired fertility.

Evaluation and treatment of infertility

Evaluation initially involves assessment of the male partner with a semen analysis and documentation of ovulatory menstrual cycles and patent fallopian tubes in the female partner. In some couples, additional testing will be indicated. This may include: anatomic assessment of the uterine cavity, evaluation of ovarian reserve by measuring serum FSH and estradiol levels in the early follicular phase of the cycle, determining ovarian antral follicle counts or random anti-Müllerian hormone (AMH) testing. Laparoscopy and/or hysteroscopy may be indicated in some patients.

Once the evaluation is complete, treatment is directed by the findings. Anovulatory or oligo-ovulatory women are treated either by correction of any underlying problem such as hyperprolactinemia or hypothyroidism or by induction of ovulation. Medications used for the induction of ovulation work by a variety of mechanisms. The most commonly used is clomiphene citrate, an estrogen partial agonist/antagonist that acts at the level of the hypothalamus and pituitary gland to block estrogenic negative feedback. This increases gonadotropin secretion. Aromatase inhibitors act to reduce circulating estrogen levels, again blocking negative feedback centrally and promoting gonadotropin production and release. Both medications require a functioning hypothalamic–pituitary–ovarian axis. Patients who are not candidates for, or who fail the prior therapies can be treated with gonadotropin (FSH +/− LH) injections.

Reproductive tract surgery to remove endometriosis or a fibroid tumor may be recommended, although medical therapy for some of these problems is also available. In the past, tubal reconstructive surgery was a mainstay of infertility treatment; where readily available, assisted reproductive techniques like *in vitro* fertilization (IVF) have virtually eliminated the need for this approach.

Treatments for male factor infertility may first address the underlying etiology directly. This may include medical or surgical therapies, such as correction of a varicocele or correction of blockage in the vas deferens. More commonly, assisted reproductive techniques are used to bypass sperm problems. Sperm can be washed, concentrated and placed directly into the intrauterine cavity using artificial insemination. The sperm source can be the woman's partner or a donor.

The widespread availability of the **assisted reproductive technologies** has revolutionized infertility treatment, making pregnancies possible under circumstances never before considered treatable. The most common treatment approach is IVF, in which multiple harvested oocytes are fertilized by spermatozoa in the laboratory. The resulting embryos are grown in the laboratory for 2–5 days, then a group of embryos is selected and transferred back into the cavity of the uterus. Standard IVF can be modified in a number of ways. Donor eggs or donor sperm can be used. In cases of severe male factor infertility, sperm can be injected directly into the oocyte cytoplasm to effect fertilization (intracytoplasmic sperm injection, ICSI). These sperm can be immotile. They can be retrieved directly from the vas deferens, epididymis, or even the testis in men with obstructive azospermia. Finally, recently developed technology allows genetic assessment of the embryos created through IVF. Using preimplantation genetic diagnosis (PGD), a single blastomere is removed from a developing blastocyst and screened for a variety of selected heritable single gene defects or for numerical chromosomal content. The results of screening can be used in selecting those embryos that will be transferred back to the uterus.

Figure 35.1 Timing of zygote or embryo division leading to different types of monozygotic twins

Ovulation age (days): 0, 1, 2, 3, 4, 5, 6, 7, 8, 9, 10, 11, 12, 13, 14

Zygote — Division occurs — 2 cell stage — Blastocyst — Chorion — Amnion — Diamniotic dichorionic

Division occurs — Blastocyst — Diamniotic monochorionic

Embryoblast — Separate primitive streaks — Duplication occurs — Monoamnionic monochorionic

Primitive streak duplicates — Conjoined twins

Figure 35.2 Transvaginal sonography shows four intrauterine gestational sacs in a pregnancy conceived through assisted reproductive techniques. Measurement of the fetal pole (crown-rump length; CRL) of the fetus present in this image dates the gestation at 6 weeks and 5 days of gestation. Some feel that chorionicity can be determined by measuring intersac distances, with a cut-off of 2 mm or greater suggesting more than 1 chorion

Yolk sac — 0.51cm — 0.38cm — Fetal pole — CRL — 0.31cm

Twins may arise from one of two mechanisms: division of a single fertilized ovum into two embryos (**"identical" or monozygotic twins**) or fertilization of two separate ova (**"fraternal" or dizygotic twins**). Either or both processes may be involved in the generation of higher numbers of fetuses. Triplets could develop from one, two or three ova; quadruplets from one, two, three or four and so on. It is exceedingly rare for a zygote to divide more than once.

The two twinning processes have very distinct origins and implications for pregnancy outcome. While all multiple gestations carry a risk of preterm delivery from early labor, monozygotic twin pregnancies carry an additional risk of placental problems, chromosomal abnormalities and fetal malformations. These can dramatically influence pregnancy outcomes.

Biology of monozygotic twinning

It is not known exactly what causes an embryo to divide to produce monozygotic twins. However, it is clear that division of the fertilized ovum at specific early stages of development is responsible for the spectrum of clinical presentations with monozygotic twinning. These stages are depicted in Fig. 35.1. Basically, the earlier the fertilized ovum divides, the more separate the twins. Cleavage prior to development of an inner cell mass will result in two placentas, two sets of membranes and two fetuses, whereas division after the embryonic disc has formed results in conjoined twins.

The most common type of monozygotic twinning arises from division during days 3–8 after fertilization. As division occurs after inner cell mass development, but before amnion or embryonic disk formation, this produces a pregnancy with two amniotic sacs and a single placenta (**diamniotic monochorionic twins**). The second most common type of monozygotic twinning results from a division of the embryo within the first 72 h after fertilization and produces a pregnancy with two amniotic sacs and two placentas (**diamniotic dichorionic twins**). Twins resulting from divisions later than day 8 after fertilization are rare. If the division occurs on or after the amnion forms on day 8 post-fertilization, both fetuses will be in the same amniotic sac (**monoamniotic monochorionic twins**). Siamese or **conjoined twins** are the rarest and arise from cleavage of the differentiating embryonic disc 13–16 days post-conception. Fraternal twins are always diamniotic dichorionic. Therefore, it is necessary to perform zygosity testing on twins with separate placentas who are suspected of being monozygous.

The Reproductive System at a Glance, Fourth Edition. Linda J. Heffner and Danny J. Schust.

78 © 2014 John Wiley & Sons, Ltd. Published 2014 by John Wiley & Sons, Ltd. Companion Website: www.ataglanceseries.com/reproduction

Etiology of dizygotic twins

Most of the spontaneously conceived multifetal pregnancies are twin gestations. The incidence of conception of twins is at least twice the rate of liveborn twins. In many cases, one of a pair of diamniotic dichorionic twins just disappears. Less often, the whole pregnancy miscarries. The frequency of monozygotic twinning is about 1 set in every 250 births and is relatively fixed in most populations. In contrast to monozygotic twinning, the incidence of dizygotic twinning varies dramatically among different populations. Dizygotic twinning is highly influenced by race and heredity. Maternal age over 40, increasing parity and infertility treatment are positively linked to dizygotic twinning.

The racial differences in dizygotic twinning are quite marked. Twinning among Asians is least common, with a rate of only 1.3 dizygotic twin births per 1000 total births in Japan. White women in the USA and the UK have rates of about 8 dizygotic twin sets per 1000 births. Black women have the highest rates of all. They range from a rate of 11 per 1000 births in the USA to 49 per 1000 in some tribes in Nigeria, or 1 in every 20 births. The influence of heredity on dizygotic twinning is carried largely through maternal lineages, with about a 2% chance of delivering twins if the mother herself is a dizygotic twin. When the father of the baby is a dizygotic twin, the rate of twinning is only 0.8%.

In developed countries, most multifetal pregnancies result from infertility treatments. Ovulation induction, *in vitro* fertilization (IVF) and other assisted reproductive techniques dramatically increase the frequency not only of twinning, but also of conceiving higher order multiple gestations (triplets, quadruplets and more); (Fig. 35.2). Table 35.1 lists recent outcome data approximating the frequency of multifetal pregnancies in the USA, dependent on the means of conception. If one uses Hellin's theorem to calculate the expected frequency of twins in Nigeria, which has the highest spontaneous twinning rate in the world, one can see the impact of infertility treatment on the higher-order multiple gestations. Hellin's theorem states that if the frequency of twinning is n in a population, then the frequency of triplets is n^2, quadruplets n^3, and so on. Using $n = 0.05$ for the Nigerian tribes, one would only expect 0.25% triplet and 0.012% quadruplet gestations. Thus, infertility treatment can increase the risk of triplets 20-fold and quadruplets 80-fold over the world's most "twiningest" people.

Although infertility treatment dramatically increases the frequency of nonidentical multiples, the rate of monozygous twinning is also double that expected in these women. A disproportionate number of these monozygotic twins are also monochorionic. Transfer of day 5 blastocysts into the uterus during IVF is associated with a higher rate of monozygotic twins than transfer of day 3 zygotes. The stimuli for monozygotic twinning following ovulation induction alone have not been identified. Elevated gonadotropins promote recruitment of more than one ovarian follicle in a given cycle and represent the single most important risk factor for dizygotic conceptions. This is most evident during infertility treatments where the use of injected gonadotropins is associated with the development of multiple ovulatory follicles. The increased rates of spontaneous twinning seen with black race, advancing maternal age, parity and heredity are also related to elevations in endogenous gonadotropins, most notably in FSH.

Pregnancy risks with multiple gestations

The inherent risk in multiple gestations depends largely on whether single or multiple placentas are present and on whether there is a shared amniotic sac. All monochorionic twins have some degree of vascular connection within the placental bed. In about 15% of monochorionic twin pregnancies, these vascular connections permit the exchange of blood between the two fetuses. When this occurs, the hemodynamics of the two twins can become so deranged that one fetus will preferentially pump extra blood into the other (**"twin–twin transfusion syndrome"**). The "donor" twin becomes anemic and produces an abnormally low amount of amniotic fluid, whereas the "recipient" twin is volume overloaded and produces excessive amounts of amniotic fluid. Fetuses in multiple gestations also have an increased risk for abnormal insertion of the umbilical cord onto the placenta. The umbilical cord typically inserts into the middle of the placental disc and is completely surrounded by a protective layer of Warton's jelly. With multiple gestations, each fetus has an increased incidence of having its cord insert along the edge of the placenta (**velamentous insertion**). Cords with velamentous insertions are not completely surrounded by Warton's jelly and can be kinked or compressed more readily than more protected cords. Such compression can result in suboptimal fetal blood flow. The umbilical cords of monoamniotic twins invariably become entangled. This leads to fetal deaths in over half of the cases.

In addition to the problems that can arise from their placentas and membranes, monozygotic twins are also at increased risk of chromosomal abnormalities and congenital malformations. Because affected twin pairs are often discordant for the abnormality, it is presumed that whatever intrauterine events caused these embryos to divide can also randomly increase the risk for disordered embryonic development.

All multiple gestations are at risk for growth restriction of one or more of the fetuses. The risk increases as the number of fetuses increases. There are many possible causes for fetal growth restriction in multiple gestations. Suboptimal perfusion of the area of placental implantation of one or more fetus can cause fetal growth restriction. Velamentous umbilical cord insertions may also cause decreased fetal perfusion and growth restriction, as can donation of blood to a co-twin in the twin–twin transfusion syndrome.

All multiple gestations are at risk for preterm labor (Chapter 37). The risk increases in parallel with increasing numbers of fetuses. Uterine distension may explain the early onset of labor in pregnancies complicated by multiple gestations; however, other nonmechanical factors may also be involved.

Table 35.1 Multifetal pregnancy rates using different infertility treatments (percentage of births)

Treatment	Twins	Triplets	Quadruplets +
None	1.2	0.015	0.00017
Aromatase inhibitors	3–4	<1	–
Clomiphene	8–10	<1	–
Gonadotropins	15	5	0.6
IVF	29	6	1

Figure 36.1 Sites of ectopic pregnancies

Isthmic (6–7% of tubal gestations)

Interstitial (~2% of tubal gestations)

Ampullary (>75% of tubal gestations)

Fimbrial (~6–7% of tubal gestations)

Ovarian (<2% of ectopic gestations)

Cervical (rare)

Abdominal (rare)

Ectopic pregnancy

Any pregnancy that implants outside of the uterine endometrial cavity is called an **ectopic pregnancy**. Despite improved diagnostic and therapeutic approaches to this disorder, ectopic pregnancy remains the most common cause of pregnancy-related maternal death in the first 12 weeks of pregnancy. A ruptured ectopic pregancy is a medical emergency. Overall, ectopic pregnancies cause 4–10% of pregnancy-related deaths with maternal hemorrhage the ultimate fatal pathway. The incidence of ectopic pregnancy rose in the USA from the 1950s through the 1990s when national recording was halted. At that time the best estimate for the incidence of ectopic pregnancy was 2 in 100 pregnancies.

The known risk factors for ectopic pregnancy focus on alterations in appropriate function of the fallopian tube. The fallopian tube is not simply a conduit for sperm and embryo passage but rather a delicate microenvironment in which cilia help to move the fluids within the fallopian tubes that transport gametes and blastocysts. Decreased ciliary movement due to exposure to elevated levels of progesterone or direct damage, ciliary and cellular destruction as the result of trauma or infectious disease, and tubal blockage from surgical interruption or scarring all promote abnormal embryo transport. Over 90% of ectopic pregnancies can be directly related to tubal pathologies. From highest to lowest risk, these include: (i) previous ectopic pregnancy; (ii) tubal sterilization or reconstructive surgery; (iii) *in utero* exposure to diethyl stilbesterol (DES); (iv) prior genital tract infection (often silent, particularly with chlamydia); (v) infertility; (vi) multiple sexual partners; (vii) cigarette smoking; (viii) young age at initiation of sexual activity; (ix) maternal age at conception of >35 years; and (x) the practice of vaginal douching. The remaining 10% of ectopic pregnancies are of unknown etiology. They may result from embryonic factors, although there is no increase in embryonic or fetal karyotypic abnormalities when ectopic gestations are compared with intrauterine gestations. Two commonly cited risk factors for ectopic pregnancy are frequently misinterpreted. The use of assisted reproductive techniques, including *in vitro* fertilization, has recently been shown to have little effect on the overall incidence of ectopic pregnancies, although the rate of the otherwise rare heterotopic pregnancy (an ectopic gestation coexisting with an intrauterine gestation) is increased. The use of an intrauterine

contraceptice device (IUD) protects against all pregnancies and thereby decreases the overall ectopic pregnancy rate. However, when pregnancy does occur with an IUD in place, the gestation is more likely to be ectopic.

Almost all ectopic pregnancies (~95%) occur in the fallopian tube (Fig. 36.1). The most common site of implantation of an ectopic gestation within the fallopian tube is in its ampullary portion. Ampullary and fimbrial ectopic gestations frequently dislodge and abort prior to rupture. As the interstitial portion of the fallopian tube has thick muscular support, interstitial ectopic gestations may develop to relatively late gestational ages prior to clinical presentation. Cervical, interstitial and heterotopic (intrauterine + ectopic) ectopic pregnancies are rare but appear to be more frequent after *in vitro* fertilization. Ovarian ectopic gestations are random events without documented risk factors. Abdominal ectopic pregnancies are exceedingly uncommon.

Miscarriage

A miscarriage is defined as a spontaneous pregnancy loss before 20 weeks' gestation; the medical term is **spontaneous abortion**. Miscarriages occur in 15% of clinically recognized pregnancies. The total number of human conceptions far exceeds the number of births. It is estimated that at least 60% of all human conceptions do not result in a viable pregnancy, with the majority of these being spontaneously lost before or shortly after an expected menses. These pregnancies can be documented by the appearance and disappearance of a pregnancy-specific hormone (human chorionic gonadotropin, hCG; Chapter 18) from the maternal bloodstream. It is clear that there is a sensitive and effective mechanism in the maternal system that can detect abnormal pregnancies and prevent survival of the overwhelming majority.

It is impossible to know the causes of those pregnancy losses that occur around the time of the expected menses, the so-called biochemical pregnancies. They probably result from a myriad of abnormalities and pregnancy loss represents the final common clinical outcome. Abnormalities may occur in the conceptus or in the microenvironment of the maternal reproductive tract at the time of conception. The latter may result from congenital or acquired anatomic defects in the uterus. They may also be caused by endocrine abnormalities that alter the

The Reproductive System at a Glance, Fourth Edition. Linda J. Heffner and Danny J. Schust.

80 © 2014 John Wiley & Sons, Ltd. Published 2014 by John Wiley & Sons, Ltd. Companion Website: www.ataglanceseries.com/reproduction

Table 36.1 Relative frequency of aberrations in chromosomally abnormal abortuses

Type	Incidence (%)
Trisomies (in order of frequencey: 16, other, 22, 21, 14, 15, 18)	52
45X	18
Triploid	17
Tetraploid	6
Unbalanced translocation	3
Other	4
Total	100

Table 36.2 Criteria defining miscarriage subtypes

Miscarriage type (known intrauterine pregnancy)	Defining criteria
Threatened abortion	Miscarriage symptoms (vaginal bleeding); no passage of POC or cervical change
Inevitable abortion	Uterine bleeding, cervix open, no POC passage
Incomplete abortion	Uterine bleeding, cervix open, incomplete passage of POCs
Complete spontaneous abortion	POCs passed, bleeding ceased, cervix closed
Missed abortion	Pregnancy demise, no miscarriage symptoms
Septic abortion	Infection of POCs prior to complete expulsion

POC, products of conception.

maturation of the ova prior to ovulation, the development of the embryo during transit to the intrauterine cavity or the growth and maturation of the endometrium as it prepares for implantation.

It is known that the **most frequent cause of overt miscarriage is a chromosomal abnormality in the conceptus**. At least 60% of miscarriages have a gross chromosomal abnormality that can be detected in the expelled fetal material. Table 36.1 lists the frequency of specific chromosomal abnormalities in miscarried material. It is usually not possible to identify a specific etiology for the remaining 40% of isolated spontaneous pregnancy losses, although some are the result of an underlying problem that can lead to recurrent pregnancy losses.

Increasing maternal age is accompanied by an increase in the frequency of chromosomal abnormalities in embryos and fetuses and in the rate of spontaneous pregnancy loss. Age-related egg abnormalities are thought to account for the majority of this effect, consistent with the dramatic rise in spontaneous pregnancy loss that is seen among mothers who are 35 or older. This effect is not noted in association with paternal age until the father of the pregnancy has reached at least 55 or 60 years. Even then, the effect is more subtle. Interestingly, an increase in the frequency of certain psychiatric disorders among offspring is associated with paternal aging. Ovum deterioration is thought to explain most of the decline in fertility after the maternal age of 40.

Most spontaneous pregnancy losses are heralded by vaginal bleeding and a fall in maternal serum hCG during the first trimester of pregnancy. These losses are subcategorized by clinical presentation as outlined in Table 36.2. During the first 12 weeks of pregnancy, maternal serum hCG normally rises with a doubling time of about 48–72 h. The hCG level will typically plateau or drop before tissue is passed in pregnancies with threatened miscarriages. Thus, it would appear that the common signaling mechanism for abnormal pregnancies may be a disruption in the expression of the hCG gene located on chromosome 19. How trisomies and other chromosomal aneuploidies produce this effect on the hCG gene is not known. Moreover, fetuses with trisomy 13, trisomy 18 and trisomy 21 (Down syndrome) can be carried to viability. It is equally puzzling how these three trisomies escape the hCG signaling surveillance. Trisomy 21 is actually associated with an increase in circulating hCG in the second trimester. This finding is used during the first trimester of pregnancy in serum screening regimens that determine Down syndrome risk.

Recurrent pregnancy loss

Because one in every six pregnancies will result in a miscarriage, it is not uncommon for a woman to experience one or more spontaneous losses during her pregnancy attempts. A woman who has had two consecutive spontaneous losses, but has never carried a pregnancy to full term, has a 35% chance of a loss in her next pregnancy. If a woman has successfully carried a pregnancy in the past, she will not reach a similar level of risk for spontaneous loss in a subsequent pregnancy until she has experienced three losses. For this reason, diagnostic work-up should be initiated in women with two losses if no successful pregnancies have occurred in the past. Clinicians may choose to wait until a third loss in patients who have had successful pregnancies. It is reasonable to consider initiating diagnostic testing at an earlier point in the clinical history among women with infertility or advanced maternal age.

Causes of recurrent pregnancy loss (recurrent miscarriage) include parental chromosome translocations; structural uterine abnormalities such as longitudinal septa and intrauterine adhesions; endocrine disorders, including luteal phase defects, polycystic ovary syndrome (PCOS), hyperprolactinemia, thyroid dysfunction and poorly controlled diabetes mellitus; autoimmune conditions such as the antiphospholipid antibody syndrome and a variety of heritable thrombophilias. Couples experiencing recurrent pregnancy losses are appropriately anxious and should be evaluated for an underlying cause in the hope that a specific intervention may prevent future spontaneous pregnancy losses.

Stillbirth

The term **stillbirth** is synonymous with **fetal death or demise**. All three terms refer to the delivery of a fetus after 20 menstrual weeks that shows no signs of life. Stillbirth rates vary widely between developed countries where the overall rate is 6–7 in 1000 births and developing countries where the rate may be as high as 30 in 1000 births. Similarly, the etiologies vary by environment and resources; in developed countries fetal growth restriction, congenital or karyotypic anomalies, and maternal medical diseases account for many stillbirths whereas pre-eclampsia, obstructed labor and infection are more common causes in less developed countries. Fetal death before the onset of labor (antepartum fetal death) is much more common than fetal death during labor or delivery (intrapartum fetal death).

There are many causes of stillbirth. **An etiology is never identified in at least 25% of stillbirths** (unexplained stillbirth) even after complete evaluation. Fetal causes for stillbirth include chromosomal and genetic abnormalities and congenital malformations. Placental causes include premature separation before delivery (abruption), hemorrhage from the fetus into the maternal circulation (fetomaternal hemorrhage) and umbilical cord complications. Other causes such as intrauterine infection and fetal growth restriction are multifactoral, often involving the mother and either placenta or fetus.

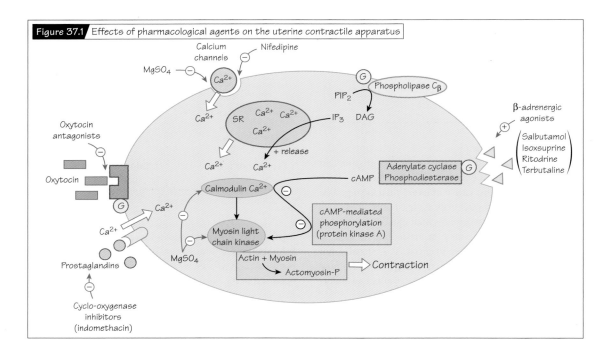

Figure 37.1 Effects of pharmacological agents on the uterine contractile apparatus

Timely onset of labor and delivery has an important role in pregnancy outcome. Both preterm and postterm births are at higher risk for poor outcomes than pregnancies delivered at term.

Preterm labor

Preterm labor is the onset of labor before 37 weeks' gestation. It is the final common pathway for a number of conditions that induce uterine contractions at a time when the uterus is normally quiescent.

Preterm labor complicates 7–10% of all pregnancies and is a very large contributor to perinatal morbidity and mortality. Although over half the cases of preterm labor occur without warning, some factors do carry an identifiable risk: multiple gestation, uterine anomalies, third trimester bleeding, intrauterine infection, excessive amniotic fluid volume, maternal smoking and a history of prior preterm delivery. There have been many unsuccessful attempts to use risk scoring, close clinical observation and home uterine contraction monitoring to predict women at high risk for preterm labor. Several biochemical markers suggest increased risk of preterm labor: raised salivary estriol, which reflects activation of the fetal hypothalamic–pituitary–adrenal axis, and cortisol-releasing hormone, which is synthesized by the placenta (Chapters 19 and 22). Fetal fibronectin is normally restricted to the fetal compartment but will appear in vaginal secretions of women who are at risk for preterm delivery. Therefore the absence of fetal fibronectin in maternal vaginal secretions is highly predictive of women who will not experience preterm labor.

Potential mechanisms for preterm labor

The normal mechanisms involved in labor (Chapter 22) predict the pathways for stimuli that start labor prematurely. For instance, intrauterine infection is associated with an elevation in the amniotic fluid levels of the cytokines interleukin-1β, interleukin-6 and tumor necro-

sis factor α (TNF-α). Products of the cyclo-oxygenase and prostaglandin pathways are also elevated in patients with intrauterine infections. Cytokines and prostaglandins act synergistically to stimulate the myometrium. Their premature elevation with intrauterine infection could activate the uterus prematurely. Recently, thrombin has been shown to be an extremely potent uterotonic agent. The increase in thrombin production that accompanies bleeding in pregnancy may cause preterm labor. Multiple gestations and excessive amniotic fluid excessively stretch the myometrial syncytium. While this may stimulate muscle activity, it is unclear how fiber stretching produces the regular, coordinated contractions of labor.

Pharmacologic interventions

In some cases of preterm labor, contractions represent an attempt by the uterus to expel the fetus from a hostile intrauterine environment. This may be the goal when premature labor accompanies intrauterine infection. It is usually not prudent to intervene by attempting to stop labor in these clinical situations. When the cause of preterm labor does not independently place the fetus in danger, pharmacologic attempts to stop the premature contractions may be used (Fig. 37.1). Several agents, called **tocolytics**, are available to inhibit premature uterine contractions. Tocolytics work by interrupting one of four processes: (i) intracellular Ca^{2+} homeostasis; (ii) myosin phosphorylation; (iii) prostaglandin synthesis; and (iv) oxytocin binding to its receptors (Fig. 37.1). Calcium ions are required for normal myometrial contractions. Magnesium sulfate ($MgSO_4$) acts as a competitive antagonist for Ca^{2+} and is a commonly used tocolytic. High extracellular magnesium concentrations inhibit Ca^{2+} entry into myometrial cells via voltage-operated channels. In addition, intracellular magnesium competes with Ca^{2+} for binding sites on calmodulin. Decreased calcium–calmodulin binding decreases the activity of myosin light chain kinase and muscle

The Reproductive System at a Glance, Fourth Edition. Linda J. Heffner and Danny J. Schust.

contraction. Nifedipine and nitrendipine are type II (dihydropyridine) calcium channel blockers. They prevent Ca^{2+} influx through the cell membrane into the myometrial cells via the voltage-operated Ca^{2+} channels. Beta-adrenergic agonists, such as ritodrine, salbutamol, isoxsuprine and terbutaline, bind to β_2-adrenergic receptors on the myometrial cell membrane, activate G proteins and increase intracellular cAMP levels. An increase in cAMP levels activates protein kinase A. Activated protein kinase A inhibits myosin light chain phosphorylation. Prostaglandins E and $F_{2\alpha}$ stimulate uterine contractions. The tocolytic, indomethacin, reduces prostaglandin production. It competitively inhibits cyclo-oxygenases that are necessary for conversion of arachidonic acid to prostaglandins. Oxytocin antagonists bind to the oxytocin receptor but do not activate it. Antagonist-binding blocks activation by the agonist oxytocin. Progesterone prophylaxis has been shown to reduce the rate of preterm birth among women with a history of spontaneous preterm delivery. The mechanism of action of the supplemental progesterone is not known.

Postterm pregnancy

Postterm pregnancy refers to a pregnancy that has extended to or beyond 42.0 weeks' gestation or 294 days from the first day of the last normal menstrual period. About 2% of pregnancies dated by first trimester ultrasound go postterm. The cause of postterm pregnancy is largely unknown. Risk factors include first pregnancy, male fetus, obesity, prior postterm pregnancy and maternal postterm birth. The latter two factors suggest that maternal genetic factors may have a role. Interesting recent data indicate that paternal genes expressed in the fetus may also be involved. Early reports that placental sulfatase deficiency and fetal anencephaly are associated with postterm pregnancy have not been corroborated.

Postterm pregnancy is linked to increased maternal and fetal risk. Labor abnormalities and cesarean deliveries increase because of fetal overgrowth and placental dysfunction. Fetal risks include stillbirth, asphyxia and birth injury from overgrowth. Management of the postterm pregnancy may include induction at 41.0 weeks' gestation or expectant management with close fetal surveillance.

Placental abnormalities

Placental abruption is defined as premature separation of the placenta prior to delivery of the fetus. Typical symptoms of placental abruption are vaginal bleeding and abdominal pain that are often accompanied by frequent prolonged uterine contractions, uterine tenderness and fetal distress. Placental abruption complicates about 1% of all births. Severe abruptions can result in stillbirth (Chapter 36).

Risk factors for placental abruption that precedes labor include maternal trauma, hypertension, uterine anomalies, inherited and acquired clotting disorders, abruption or pre-eclampsia in a prior pregnancy, poor fetal growth, cocaine use, cigarette smoking and acute intrauterine infection. Rupture of the fetal membranes, either prior to the onset of labor or during labor in the presence of excess amniotic fluid, is also associated with increased risk for placental abruption.

Most commonly, the cause of the placental separation is the rupture of maternal vessels in the decidua basalis next to the placental villi. Rupture of vessels may result from acute trauma, high intravascular pressures or from chronic inflammation and/or necrosis. Maternal blood infiltrates into the decidua and lifts it off of the placenta. The resulting hematoma may stay small or it may enlarge to completely separate the placenta from the uterine wall. Thrombin, an important component of the clotting cascade, is released from the decidua in response to the local hypoxia that accompanies abruption. Thrombin is a very potent uterotonic agent; its release likely produces the exaggerated uterine activity seen with abruption. Thrombin also induces expression of inflammatory cytokines, leading to additional vascular disruption. The detached portion of the placenta cannot exchange gases or deliver nutrients for the duration of the pregnancy. Pregnancy outcome is largely dependent on the size of the separation.

The amount of vaginal bleeding from a placental abruption is not a good indicator of the extent of the separation because some or all of the bleeding can be concealed within the uterus. In cases of abruption severe enough to kill the fetus, maternal disseminated intravascular coagulation can develop due to consumption of available clotting factors by the massive amounts of released thrombin. Management of placental abruption depends on severity and gestational age.

Placenta previa refers to the presence of placental tissue overlying or extremely close to the internal os of the cervix. It occurs in 5–6% of first trimester gestations; however, placental migration away from the cervix results in an incidence of 0.5% in the third trimester. The diagnosis is made by ultrasound examination of the pregnancy within the uterus. Risk factors for placenta previa include prior cesarean delivery and uterine curettage, advancing maternal age and parity, cigarette smoking, multiple gestation and male fetal gender. Conditions associated with placenta previa include placenta accreta, velamentous umbilical cord insertion, vasa previa and abnormal fetal lie. **Placenta accreta** occurs when the placenta traverses the decidua and invades the myometrium. Velamentous insertion of the umbilical cord occurs when the fetal blood vessels do not insert on the disc of the placenta, presumably as a result of abnormal placental migration. Vasa previa is a rare condition in which the umbilical blood vessels insert onto the fetal membranes instead of the placenta and a fetal vessel lies over the internal os of the cervix.

Placenta previa is thought to occur when an embryo fails to implant in the upper segment of the uterus. Reasons for the abnormal implantation include scarring of the uterus from cesarean deliveries, uterine curettage and prior pregnancies, a need for increased placental surface area to compensate for a reduction in uteroplacental nutrient or oxygen delivery such as occurs with maternal smoking or multiple gestation, and delayed implantation associated with later fertilization in male embryos. An abnormal fetal lie may result from the large volume of placenta in the lower portion of the uterine cavity with a placenta previa.

Abnormal fetal lie and presentation

The term "lie" refers to the orientation of the fetus in the uterus. By far the most common fetal lie is longitudinal. Transverse lie means the fetus is lying sideways in the uterus. Occasionally, the fetal and maternal axes will cross at a 45° angle, forming an oblique lie. Oblique lies are unstable and will usually convert to a longitudinal lie in labor. Only longitudinal lies can safely be delivered vaginally.

Presentation refers to the fetal part that is in closest proximity to the birth canal. The most common fetal presentation is head-down (cephalic or vertex); 95% of fetuses are vertex at term. The second most common presentation is breech, in which the fetal legs or buttocks are just above the cervix. A shoulder typically presents when the fetus is lying transverse.

The major risk factor for abnormal fetal lie and presentation is prematurity. Other risk factors include fetal malformations, congenital neuromuscular disorders, multiple gestation, uterine malformations and high maternal parity (number of prior births).

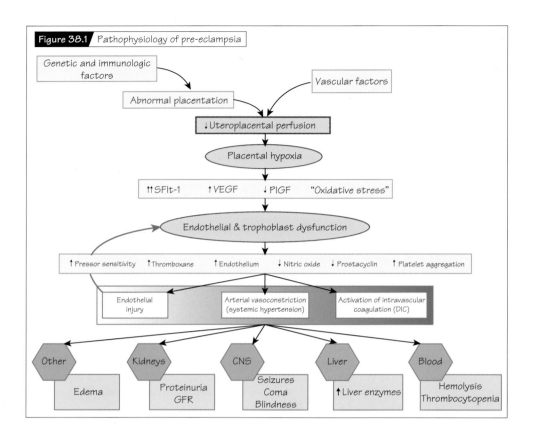

Figure 38.1 Pathophysiology of pre-eclampsia

Clinical spectrum of pre-eclampsia

Pre-eclampsia is a unique disorder found only in human pregnancies. **Historically, pre-eclampsia has been defined as the triad of hypertension, proteinuria and edema** in a pregnant woman. **Eclampsia** is the occurrence of seizures that cannot be attributed to another cause in a patient with pre-eclampsia. Pre-eclampsia typically occurs in the third trimester of pregnancy, although some cases manifest earlier. Although many patients with pre-eclampsia demonstrate the classic triad, it is now clear that the disorder is really a spectrum of clinical signs and symptoms that accompany microvascular changes in multiple organ systems (Fig. 38.1). The disorder has so many presentations that it has been called the "great imitator." Central nervous system involvement can result in severe headaches, visual changes, seizures, stroke and blindness. Renal involvement is almost always present and can manifest as proteinuria, oliguria or renal failure. Edema can accumulate in many sites, including the feet, hands, face and lungs. Hemoconcentration, thrombocytopenia and intravascular hemolysis are common signs of hematologic involvement. Hepatic dysfunction often accompanies hematologic changes and produces a group of clinical findings known as **HELLP syndrome** (**h**emolysis, **e**levated **l**iver function tests, **l**ow **p**latelets). Patients with HELLP will often develop vague epigastric pain resulting from liver involvement which may be mistaken for heartburn, gallbladder disease or the flu by an unsuspecting health care provider.

The overall incidence of pre-eclampsia in the obstetric population is 5–8%; the absolute number depends on the proportion of patients at increased risk. Risk factors for developing pre-eclampsia include the primigravid state (first pregnancy), multiple gestation, diabetes, pre-existing hypertension, a long interval between pregnancies, pre-eclampsia in a previous pregnancy, a family history of pre-eclampsia, hydatidiform mole, and inherited and acquired clotting disorders (e.g., protein S and protein C deficiencies and antiphospholipid antibodies). There is considerable overlap between the risk factors for pre-eclampsia and those for fetal growth restriction (FGR). Indeed, the presence of FGR may be the first sign of impending pre-eclampsia and women with pre-eclampsia are at risk for delivering a growth-restricted baby.

Left untreated, pre-eclampsia can be a highly morbid and even fatal disease. The ultimate treatment for the condition is delivery of the pregnancy. This is so effective a therapy that all deranged physiology will revert to normal after delivery provided that no permanent tissue damage has occurred. If the mother is medically supported through a timely delivery and postpartum recovery, her kidneys will begin to make urine again, blood will clot and seizures will stop. In spite of its potential for a 100% cure with proper diagnosis and treatment, pre-eclampsia remains one of the leading causes of maternal death in both developed and developing countries.

Potential mechanisms in pre-eclampsia pathogenesis

It is clear that placental abnormalities are central to the pathogenesis of pre-eclampsia. Delivery cures pre-eclampsia and hydatidiform

The Reproductive System at a Glance, Fourth Edition. Linda J. Heffner and Danny J. Schust.

Figure 38.2 (a) Non-preeclamptic placentation

Syncytiotrophoblast
Floating villae
Intervillous space
Anchoring villae
Fetal vessels
Villous cytotrophoblast
Vascular endothelia
Endovascular cytotrophoblast
Interstitial cytotrophoblast
Extravillous cytotrophoblast

Figure 38.2 (b) Preeclamptic placentation

Syncytiotrophoblast
Floating villae
Intervillous space
Anchoring villae
Fetal vessels
Villous cytotrophoblast
Vascular endothelia
Endovascular cytotrophoblast
Interstitial cytotrophoblast
Extravillous cytotrophoblast

mole, a form of gestational trophoblast disease characterized by placental overgrowth but no fetal development (Chapter 45), predisposes to the disease. It was originally thought that the placenta secreted a toxin that caused pre-eclampsia and the disorder was appropriately called "**toxemia**." While no unique toxins have been identified in the circulation of patients with pre-eclampsia, abnormal concentrations of specific metabolites are found in many of these patients. Circulating thromboxane, a vasoconstricting prostaglandin, is elevated while nitric oxide production is subnormal. A number of other factors, including a soluble form of a vascular endothelial growth factor (VEGF) receptor (sVEGFR-1 or sFlt-1), placental growth factor (PLGF) and soluble endoglin (sENG), a circulating receptor for transforming growth factor β (TGF-β), have been shown to be markedly different in the serum of pregnant women weeks or months before the symptoms of pre-eclampsia manifest. Unfortunately, the test accuracies of these markers are inadequate to predict pre-eclampsia in clinical practice.

There are many unproven but enticing theories about the etiology and pathogenesis of pre-eclampsia. It is likely that there are several initiators of the disease that ultimately converge in a final common pathway. Examination of the small blood vessels in the uteri of women with pre-eclampsia often reveals a failure of the invading trophoblast to remodel the spiral arteries (Fig. 38.2). There are several explanations for why the cytotrophoblast might fail to invade these vessels including abnormal immune activation or genetic predisposition. Cytotrophoblast differentiation into an invasive phenotype is accompanied by increased production of VEGF and PLGF, both proangiogenic factors. Placentas from pre-eclamptic pregnancies secrete increased amounts of sFlt-1, the soluble antagonist to VEGF, and sENG; both are antiangiogenic factors.

Abnormal immune activation that inhibits trophoblast invasion of maternal blood vessels could explain why pre-eclampsia is most common when a woman is exposed to paternal antigens for the first time: a first pregnancy or, in a multigravid woman, the initial pregnancy with a new partner. Loss of immune tolerance over time would also explain why a long interval between pregnancies is a risk factor for developing pre-eclampsia. Abnormal activation of the immune system underlies other autoimmune diseases, such as systemic lupus erythematosus, that carry an increased risk for pre-eclampsia. Some women with pre-eclampsia have activating autoantibodies to the angiotensin II receptor that inhibit trophoblast invasiveness *in vitro*.

Specific genetic abnormalities may be involved in the pathophysiology of pre-eclampsia. Women who carry a mutation in the complement receptor CR-1 have an increased risk for pre-eclampsia as do women carrying a specific polymorphism for plasminogen activator inhibitor type 1. Pre-existing insulin resistance confers an increased risk. The fact that a family history of pre-eclampsia increases a woman's risk for the disease indicates that there may be many additional genetic predispositions to the disease.

A mismatch between fetal and placental demands and the maternal ability to meet them may also cause pre-eclampsia and would explain risk factors such as multiple gestation, maternal vascular disease and hypercoagulable states. Proponents of this theory propose that the undernourished fetus sends signals to the mother to increase perfusion of the placenta. If the mother cannot compensate in response to these initial signals, the fetus sends more urgent signals. Pre-eclampsia would theoretically result from the effects of excessive signals. As an example, hypoxia has been shown to increase the production of sFlt-1 by trophoblast cells. Increased sFlt-1 may be part of the pathogenesis of pre-eclampsia.

While the initiating placental abnormality is unclear, the final common pathway for pre-eclampsia is known to be **endothelial dysfunction and injury**. The vascular endothelium normally functions to prevent microcoagulation and to modulate vascular tone. Vascular injury results in coagulation and alters the response of the underlying vascular smooth muscle to vasoactive substances. Often, substances that act as vasodilators on an intact endothelium will cause vasoconstriction of damaged endothelium. In pre-eclampsia, endothelial dysfunction can solely explain the basic triad: hypertension (vasospasm), edema (capillary leak) and proteinuria (renal cell damage secondary to hypoperfusion). Experiments in animal models indicate that excess sFlt-1 can directly produce some of the organ dysfunction seen in pre-eclampsia. What remains inexplicable is why only a few, but not all, of the signs and symptoms of pre-eclampsia will appear in any given patient.

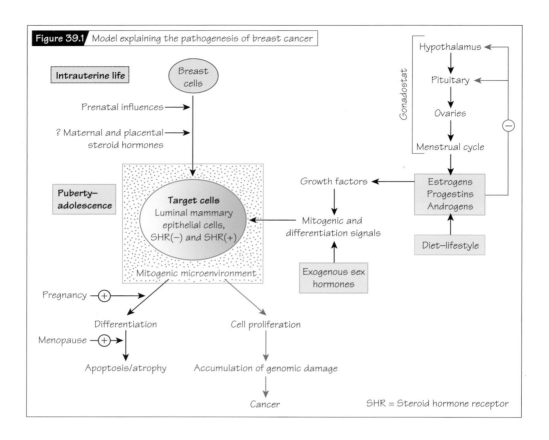

Figure 39.1 Model explaining the pathogenesis of breast cancer

Intrauterine life

Breast cells

Prenatal influences →

? Maternal and placental steroid hormones →

Puberty–adolescence

Target cells
Luminal mammary epithelial cells, SHR(−) and SHR(+)

Mitogenic microenvironment

Pregnancy —⊕→

Menopause —⊕→

Differentiation

Apoptosis/atrophy

Cell proliferation

Accumulation of genomic damage

Cancer

Growth factors ←

Mitogenic and differentiation signals

Exogenous sex hormones

Gonadostat

Hypothalamus

Pituitary

Ovaries

Menstrual cycle

Estrogens Progestins Androgens

Diet–lifestyle

⊖

SHR = Steroid hormone receptor

Common benign breast diseases

Breast complaints are common in women and most diseases of the breast (96%) are nonmalignant. Histologic subcategorization of breast masses, based upon cellular proliferation and the presence or absence of hyperplasia, divides these lesions into three subgroups. **Nonproliferative lesions** include simple and complex cysts. While most cystic lesions do not increase breast cancer risk, complex cysts containing solid and cystic components on ultrasound have increased malignant potential. **Proliferative lesions without atypia** include fibroadenomas, simple ductal and intraductal hyperplasia, sclerosing adenosis and papillomas. The latter are often associated with unilateral nipple discharge. All of these solid lesions increase breast cancer risk with a relative risk (RR) of 1.6–1.9. **Proliferative lesions with atypia (atypical hyperplasia)** can be of ductal or lobular origin. They increase the risk of breast cancer 3.7–5.3-fold.

Other common breast disorders include mastitis, cyclical breast pain and nipple discharge. Mastitis affects 3–10% of lactating women and typically presents as unilateral breast pain and high fever. Cyclical breast pain is often related to the hormonal changes of the menstrual cycle. Risk of malignancy after normal exam and imaging of the painful breast is very low. Most women of reproductive age can express discharge from their nipples. However, unilateral discharge, the presence of blood, age greater than 40 and association with a breast mass are concerning and require additional testing.

Breast cancer

Breast cancer is the most common malignancy in women. In addition to occuring almost exclusively in women, it is also a disease of aging. The lifetime risk of developing breast cancer (1 in 8) is largely concentrated in the perimenopausal and postmenopausal years. Risk in the 30-year-old is 1 in 2525, that in a 45-year-old 1 in 93 and that in a 65-year-old 1 in 17. Older women tend to underestimate their risk and many women under 50 years of age grossly overestimate their risk. Consequently, these two groups of women misjudge the benefits of breast cancer screening programs.

Breast cancer can arise anywhere in the mammary gland. Tumors are typically classified by their cells of origin: lobular or ductal. Ductal carcinomas account for 85% of breast cancers and can be either noninvasive (intraductal) or infiltrating. Those ductal carcinomas that are histologically confined by the basement membrane of the duct are called intraductal carcinomas or ductal carcinoma *in situ* (DCIS). DCIS is considered a precursor lesion to invasive carcinoma. At least 33% of these lesions will progress to invasive cancer within 5 years.

Once the basement membrane of the duct is breached, an infiltrating carcinoma has developed. The most common type of invasive carcinoma is ductal carcinoma, which accounts for 79% of invasive carcinomas. The next most common type is lobular carcinoma. These lesions arise from the terminal ductules of the alveoli and comprise approximately 10% of invasive breast cancers. Less common types of infiltrat-

The Reproductive System at a Glance, Fourth Edition. Linda J. Heffner and Danny J. Schust.

Table 39.1 Determinants of breast cancer risk

Factor	Relative risk
Family history of breast cancer	
First-degree relative	1.8
Premenopausal first-degree relative	3.0
Postmenopausal first-degree relative	1.5
Premenopausal first-degree relative (bilateral breast cancer)	9.0
Postmenopausal first-degree relative (bilateral breast cancer)	4.0–5.4
Menstrual history	
Menarche before age 12	1.7–3.4
Menarche after age 17	0.3
Menopause before age 45	0.5–0.7
Menopause at age 45–54	1.0
Menopause after age 55	1.5
Menopause after age 55 with more than 40 menstrual years	2.5–5.0
Oophorectomy before age 35	0.4
Anovulatory menstrual cycles	2.0–4.0
Pregnancy history	
Term pregnancy before age 20	0.4
First term pregnancy at age 20–34	1.0
First term pregnancy after age 35	1.5–4.0
Nulliparous patient	1.3–4.0
Histologic risk factors	
Atypical ductal hyperplasia	1.3–4.5
Atypical lobular hyperplasia	4.0
Lobular carcinoma *in situ*	5.4–12.0
Other	
Affluent vs. poor	2.0
Jewish vs. non-Jewish	2.0
Western hemisphere	1.5
Cold climate	1.5
Obesity + hypertension + diabetes	3.0
Moderate alcohol intake	1.3

ing carcinomas include medullary carcinomas, mucinous (colloid) carcinomas and Paget disease. Paget disease is a special subtype of infiltrating ductal carcinoma localized to a main lactiferous duct. In Paget disease, eczematous changes develop in the nipple and areola overlying the affected duct. These skin changes are often the first sign of disease although the cancer may have been present for some time.

Breast cancer metastasizes first to the regional axillary lymph nodes. The most frequent distant metastatic sites are bone, liver, lung, pleura and brain. Patients with histologically negative axillary nodes have a much higher likelihood of survival than do patients with positive nodes. The ultimate prognosis for the disease depends on the size of the tumor, the number of involved lymph nodes and whether or not lymphovascular invasion (LVI) is present.

Treatment of invasive breast cancer is typically multimodal, but ultimately depends on the stage of the disease at the time of diagnosis. Surgical options include a modified radical mastectomy or lumpectomy with local irradiation. Ipsilateral axillary lymph node dissection is also typically performed. Women with positive lymph nodes will usually receive additional antineoplastic chemotherapy. Those with negative nodes will receive adjuvant chemotherapy if they have large primary tumors or LVI, because both confer a high risk of tumor recurrence. Tamoxifen is a medication with estrogenic and antiestrogenic properties; it is the most widely used endocrine therapy for breast cancer. Before employing endocrine therapy, it is important to know the estrogen and progesterone receptor status of the tumor because only receptor-positive tumors predictably respond to medications like tamoxifen.

Treatment of DCIS is controversial and includes mastectomy or wide local excision plus irradiation. Recurrence rates following excision plus radiation are approximately 10%; half of these are invasive.

Epidemiology of breast cancer

The epidemiology of breast cancer in women suggests that it is an endocrine disorder related to prolonged exposure to ovarian hormones (Fig. 39.1). Ovarian hormones have been shown to increase the mitotic activity of mammary cells in culture. In addition to the factors listed in Table 39.1, hormonal treatment in the form of postmenopausal hormone replacement therapy may contribute to a higher lifetime risk of breast cancer.

There are also large ethnic and geographic differences in the prevalence of breast cancer. Asian women born and raised in Asia have one-fifth the risk of developing breast cancer that American women have. The risk rises toward the American level if Asians live in the USA for two or more generations, suggesting an environmental or lifestyle influence on the disease. Even within a single large country, breast cancer incidence and mortality rates can vary by location. In more affluent areas, breast cancer rates are elevated. This may be related to delayed child-bearing among more affluent and better educated women. The association of alcohol intake with increased breast cancer risk suggests there is an environmental influence on its development.

Familial breast cancer

About 10% of breast cancer is familial. The clustering of breast cancers with ovarian cancers in many familial cases led to the discovery of two genes, *BRCA1* and *BRCA2*. Individuals with germ-line mutations in these genes are at high risk for the development of specific cancers. Current evidence indicates that 25% of inherited cases of breast cancer result from mutations involving *BRCA1* and *BRCA2*. Both *BRCA1* and *BRCA2* are tumor suppressor genes and mutation in a single allele of either gene confers an increased cancer risk. The ethnic and geographic distributions of *BRCA1* and *BRCA2* are discussed in more detail in Chapter 42.

Molecular biology of sporadic (nonfamilial) breast cancer

Molecular studies have identified several genetic loci that are frequently abnormal in breast cancer specimens but not in normal breast tissues. The most commonly encountered abnormalities involve the oncogenes, *ERBB2* and c-*myc*, the tumor suppressor gene *TP53*, and telomerase. Both oncogenes are amplified or overexpressed in about 30% of breast cancers; telomerase activity is elevated in 80–90%. Breast tissue with *ERBB2* abnormalities appears to be resistant to the effects of the antiestrogen tamoxifen but more sensitive to standard chemotherapeutic agents. *TP53* abnormalities interfere with normal apoptosis, thereby making affected tumors more resistant to chemotherapy and radiation therapy. Like most malignancies, breast cancer probably results from the effects of environmental triggers on genetically susceptible tissues.

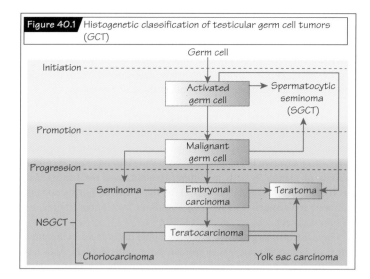

Figure 40.1 Histogenetic classification of testicular germ cell tumors (GCT)

Testicular cancer is the most common malignancy in men in the 20–40-year age group. The germ-cell tumors (GCTs) are the most prevalent type of testicular cancer. Their incidence has risen over the past two decades, as has the most prevalent risk factor for GCT, an undescended testis (cryptorchidism), suggesting that numbers of men afflicted with testicular cancer will continue to rise for the foreseeable future.

Unlike ovarian tumors, which are likely to arise from the epithelium covering the gland, 90% of primary testicular tumors arise from intratubular germ cells. Histologically, there are six distinct types of GCT. Five of these occur in young men and one is seen exclusively in older men (Fig. 40.1). The five subtypes seen in young men include **seminoma**, **choriocarcinoma**, **endodermal sinus tumor** (yolk sac carcinoma), **embryonal carcinoma** and **teratomas**, both benign and malignant. **Spermatocytic seminomas** are typically seen in men over 50 and are quite rare. The germ cells of origin in GCT affecting young and old men are distinct and appear to be at different stages of maturation. The associated tumors therefore have distinct neoplastic behaviors.

All GCTs of young men arise from spermatogonial cells. The five tumors that develop from this single precursor cell type are quite heterogeneous and several exhibit embryonal-like differentiation. Prognosis and treatment depends upon whether GCTs are pure seminomas (SGCTs) or mixed cell tumors (nonseminomas, NSGCTs). Seminomas have a homogeneous germ-cell morphology. Nonseminomas have features of embryonal cells and can mimic the histogenesis of the very early embryo. Embryonal carcinoma is the most primitive, or pluripotent, of the NSGCTs. It can progress along extraembryonic lines as choriocarcinoma or yolk sac carcinoma, or along embryonic lines as a teratoma. Individual tumors can contain a mixture of any of the histologic subtypes.

About 80% of GCTs secrete tumor markers that can be detected in the serum. Tumors with yolk sac components typically secrete alpha fetoprotein (AFP), an embryonic protein normally produced by the yolk sac during development. Other NSGCTs can also secrete AFP but seminomas do not. Human chorionic gonadotropin (hCG) is typically secreted by choriocarcinomas; however, small amounts of hCG production have been found in SGCTs as well as NSGCTs. The distribution of these two markers by specific cell types suggests the associated tumors arise from precursors at different levels of differentiation. AFP is a very primitive marker of embryonal differentiation whereas hCG represents trophoblastic differentiation. A third marker, placental-like alkaline phosphatase (PLAP), is found in carcinoma *in situ* (CIS) and about 50% of seminomas. Clinical paradigms using serum levels of AFP and hCG have been developed to assist in the diagnosis and staging of GCT.

Most GCTs are diagnosed at an early tumor stage when the tumor is confined to the testis. Serum screening, physical exam and testicular ultrasounds are useful in identifying early tumors in patients at high risk for GCT, such as formerly cryptorchid men and intersex individuals who keep their gonads. Men who present with solid testicular masses are usually treated by radical orchidectomy (removal of the testis). When GCT metastasizes, it typically spreads unilaterally to the para-aortic nodes. Distant metastases are generally found only in tumors with trophoblastic components.

Like gestational trophoblast disease in women (Chapter 45), GCT has a very high cure rate. Virtually all patients with early stage disease can expect to be cured. Initial treatment of stage I disease involves removal of the affected testes, followed by either retroperitoneal lymph node dissection, a short course of adjuvant chemotherapy or close surveillance. Even metastatic disease responds to chemotherapy with cure rates in excess of 90%.

Leydig cell tumors are a very rare form of testicular cancer (1–3%) and are associated with isosexual precocious puberty (Chapter 28). **Gonadal stromal tumors** (sex cord-stromal tumors) include both Sertoli–Leydig cell and granulosa-theca cell tumors. They are extraordinarily rare in boys and men and are associated with phenotypic feminization.

Epidemiology of GCT

The single largest risk factor for GCT is cryptorchidism (Chapter 26). It is estimated that 2–3% of cryptorchid men will develop GCT, a relative risk 5–10 times that of the general population. GCT disproportionately affects white men of European descent and is uncommon in African and Asian men, independent of where they currently reside. Familial cases are also common. Pedigree analyses suggest that a single dominant gene with low penetrance is involved in these cases.

The strong developmental association of cryptorchidism with hormonal abnormalities suggests that fetal or neonatal endocrine imbalances may be involved in the initiation of GCT. The higher incidence of testicular cancer, cryptorchidism and hypospadias seen among the sons of women who were treated with the synthetic estrogen diethylstilbestrol (DES) may provide mechanistic insights. Overexposure to estrogens during fetal development may provide activation (Fig. 40.1). Increased levels of maternal estrogen can suppress the fetal pituitary production of follicle-stimulating hormone (FSH) through negative feedback. Less FSH leads to reduced Sertoli cell multiplication and lower levels of Müllerian-inhibiting substance (MIS). Increased estrogens may also impair Leydig cell function, thus decreasing local androgen production and inhibiting testicular descent. MIS has been implicated as necessary for both normal descent of the testes and normal differentiation of fetal gonocytes into early spermatogonia. Over the past 20 years, maternal estrogen ingestion in the form of phytoestrogens

The Reproductive System at a Glance, Fourth Edition. Linda J. Heffner and Danny J. Schust.

Figure 40.2 Hypothetical scheme of human testicular germ cell tumor development

Type of germ cells / DNA characteristics	Primordial germ cells	Spermatogonia	Binucleated dysplastic germ cells	Atypical germ cells	Seminoma cells	Cells of embryonal carcinoma
Ploidy (chromosome)	Euploid (46 XY)	Euploid (46 XY)	Euploid/ aneuploid	Aneuploid (70–80 XY)	Aneuploid (70–80 XY)	Aneuploid (55–65 XY)
Evolution of germ cell tumors			Activation 1		Activation 2	

Figure 40.3 Histology of testicular seminoma-diffuse sheets of clear tumor cells with prominent nucleoli separated by fibrous trabeculae with intense lymphocytic infiltration

(soya) and chemical pollutants with estrogenic activity has increased, as has the incidence of both cryptorchidism and GCT.

Exposure of the cryptorchid testis to high temperatures may also have a role in the development of GCT, as the maturation of gonocytes to early spermatogonia is significantly inhibited in abdominal testes. Still, maldescended testes that have been restored to the scrotum in infancy or childhood do retain an increased lifetime risk of GCT, as does the contralateral testis in cases of unilateral cryptorchidism. Heat exposure cannot be solely responsible.

Molecular biology of GCT

Because all GCTs have a sex chromosome constitution of XY, all tumors must originate in germ cells prior to the first meiotic division. These tumors are often aneuploid. Most common is a near triploid autosome content. Almost all GCTs exhibit multiple copies of chromosome 12p, either as one or more copies of i(12p) or as tandemly duplicated segments of 12p on marker chromosomes. These findings have led to the following model of tumorigenesis in GCT.

The precursor cell for GCT is the pachytene spermatocyte. These are the final premeiotic spermatogonial cells and therefore contain a 4n DNA content (Chapters 4 and 8). The homologous autosomes within these cells are paired as bivalents and the sex chromosomes are aligned. These chromosomes will cross-over and segregate as they progress to metaphase 1. The process of crossing-over requires activation of specific genes to repair the resulting open chromosomal ends. If the repair mechanisms fail, the affected spermatocyte degenerates. A meiosis stage cell with a defective repair mechanism is rescued from death only by the initiation of a new program for mitotic division. Such a proliferation is neoplastic. In the spermatocyte, the aberrant chromatid exchange event that initiates the new cell cycle must involve a locus on p12, given that it is almost uniformly abnormal in GCT. Aberrations in the p12 gene product appear to rescue the cell from death. Initiation of another round of DNA replication in the improperly repaired cell will lead to a tetraploid cell with an i(p12) or amplified p12. Because the initial repair defect remains, the cell is genetically unstable and more susceptible to additional chromosomal changes, such as nondisjunction, mutation and microdeletion.

It is not clear whether all GCTs derive from a single cell that has undergone malignant transformation (clonal expansion) or whether tumorigenesis can be multifocal. An alternative, but related, theory for GCT development hypothesizes that a subset of gonocytes experiences "activation 1," during which the gonocytes become binucleated or multinucleated spermatogonia (Fig. 40.2). Nuclear fusion occurs in some of these abnormal spermatogonia and they become tetraploid cells. These aneuploid cells then receive a "second hit" or "activation 2." As a result, they lose specific genes or chromosomes that are important for tumor suppression. The clonality or multifocality of a given tumor might then depend on the nature of specific activating factors.

Regardless of how these cells undergo malignant transformation, it is clear that tumorigenesis can occur in infancy or even prenatally, perhaps as early as during testicular differentiation. Testicular CIS has been found in both fetal and neonatal testes. It is a polyploid noninvasive precursor to GCT that shares its aneuploidy and 12p amplifications. As the peak incidence of frankly invasive carcinoma occurs 2–3 decades after precursor lesions, GCT appears to have a very long latency, which supports the second hit or activation theory for the development of GCT. Early hormonal imbalances, particularly androgen exposure at puberty, may also have a role in the development of GCT, perhaps through the "activation 2" step.

In contrast to GCT in young men, the spermatocytic seminomas seen in older men are more indolent and slow growing. Spermatocytic seminomas appear to arise from mature spermatogonia and not from spermatogonial stem cells, which may explain their less aggressive behavior. The molecular basis for such different biological behaviors may rely on imprinting (discussed further in Chapter 45).

41 Diseases of the prostate

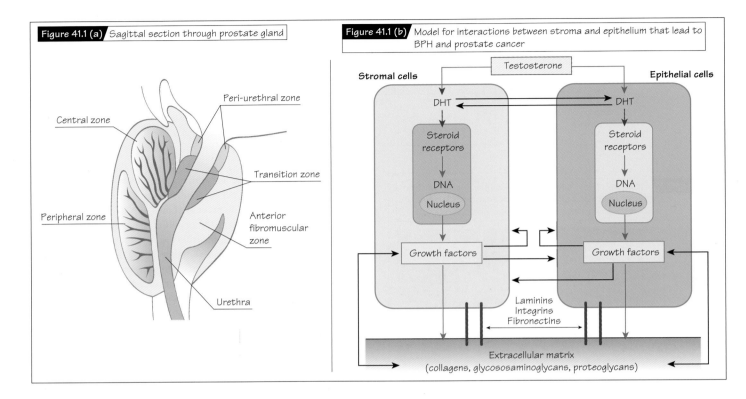

Figure 41.1 (a) Sagittal section through prostate gland

Peri-urethral zone
Central zone
Transition zone
Peripheral zone
Anterior fibromuscular zone
Urethra

Figure 41.1 (b) Model for interactions between stroma and epithelium that lead to BPH and prostate cancer

Testosterone
Stromal cells
Epithelial cells
DHT
DHT
Steroid receptors
Steroid receptors
DNA
DNA
Nucleus
Nucleus
Growth factors
Growth factors
Laminins
Integrins
Fibronectins
Extracellular matrix
(collagens, glycososaminoglycans, proteoglycans)

Benign prostatic hyperplasia

The prostate is the organ of the body most frequently afflicted by disease in males over 50 years of age. The single most common pathologic process is benign prostatic hyperplasia (BPH). At least 70% of 70-year-old men develop BPH; 40% develop some symptom of bladder outflow obstruction.

Epidemiology and symptoms

Age is a risk factor for BPH. Data suggesting that black race puts men at increased risk appear to be poorly controlled for socioeconomic status and access to health care.

BPH causes urethral obstruction severe enough to warrant medical intervention in about 30% of elderly men. Interestingly, the overall size of the prostate does not correlate with either the presence or the severity of outflow obstruction. The fibromuscular hypertrophy that occurs with BPH can partially denervate prostatic and surrounding tissues, leading to urethral irritation and producing frequency and urgency of micturition, urge incontinence and nocturia.

BPH is characterized by a gradual increase in both the glandular and fibromuscular tissue in the periurethral and transition zones of the prostate that surround the urethra at its origin from the bladder and midsegment, respectively. Nodular hyperplasia is the characteristic microscopic change of BPH. It involves cellular hyperplasia plus associated changes in the architecture of the ducts and acini. Nodular hyperplasia in the transition zone is characterized by large amounts of glandular tissue that arise through budding and branching of pre-existing ducts. This latter type of hyperplastic proliferation is a highly unusual finding in adult human tissues, whether normal or diseased.

It is felt that this anomalous development results from a reversion of the tissue to more embryonic behaviors.

Pathogenesis

Transition and central zones of the adult prostate gland seem to be of Wolffian duct derivation while the peripheral zone arises from the urogenital sinus (Chapter 6). These diverse embryological origins may explain why **BPH occurs within the transition and central zones** while prostatic adenocarcinoma originates within the peripheral zone (Fig. 41.1a).

The prostate glandular tissue is unique among the internal genitalia in that it requires dihydrotestosterone (DHT) for normal embryologic development and for maintenance. Testosterone acts as a prohormone. It is converted locally to the more potent androgen DHT by 5α-reductase. DHT potency rests on the higher affinity of the prostatic nuclear androgen receptor for DHT than for testosterone (see Chapter 2).

Differentiation and growth of prostatic epithelium is dependent on androgen-sensitive factors produced in the underlying stroma (embryological mesenchyme). Candidate growth factors increase mitosis in prostatic epithelial cells *in vitro* and include epidermal growth factor (EGF), insulin-like growth factors (IGFs) and basic fibroblast growth factor (bFGF). Expression of bFGF increases in BPH.

Development of BPH requires a normally functioning testis and 5α-reductase. Individuals lacking 5α-reductase have a vestigial prostate and never develop BPH or prostate cancer. Men with BPH have raised 5α-reductase activity and possibly an increase in prostate androgen receptors, making the "aging" prostate more susceptible to androgen stimulation. There may be a protective role for estrogens in BPH.

The Reproductive System at a Glance, Fourth Edition. Linda J. Heffner and Danny J. Schust.

Estradiol production slowly increases in older men when the testes become less responsive to luteinizing hormone (LH) so that more LH is required to maintain androgen production. High LH levels disproportionately stimulate estrogen production. Elevated circulating estrogens increase hepatic sex hormone-binding globulin (SHBG) synthesis and elevations in SHBG reduce concentrations of free testosterone in the circulation. This decreases the amount of testosterone available to be converted to DHT in the prostatic stroma.

It is believed that the clinical symptoms of BPH are not caused simply by an increase in urethral resistance due to enlargement of the prostate. Many of the symptoms formerly thought to be secondary to BPH are related to age-related bladder dysfunction, generally referred to as lower urinary tract symptoms (LUTS).

Treatment of BPH and LUTS

Medical treatment is now the preferred treatment for BPH. It focuses on shrinking the prostate using 5α-reductase inhibitors and on symptomatically treating obstructive symptoms with α-adrenergic agents. The latter are effective because of the large proportion of smooth muscle containing adrenergic receptors in BPH. Because the symptoms of BPH are also caused by bladder dysfunction, antimuscarinic agents that act on bladder muscle receptors are used in select cases.

Surgical treatment of BPH includes transurethral prostatectomy (TURP), treatment of BPH tissue using laser technology and microwave therapy to the prostate.

Prostate cancer

Prostate cancer (PCa) is the most common noncutaneous malignancy in the USA and Europe. It will certainly grow in frequency as the population ages. Autopsy series have consistently found incidental PCa in 30–80% of older men.

Epidemiology

Risk factors for PCa include age, race, positive family history, dietary fat intake and circulating hormone concentrations. African-American men who consume a high-fat diet are at the highest risk for PCa. Asian men residing in the Far East who subsist on a low-fat diet carry the lowest risk. Changes in geography or eating habits profoundly modify these background racial differences. Plasma androgen concentrations at the high end of normal increase PCa risk, as do SHBG or estrogen concentrations at the lower end of the normal range.

As with most malignancies, PCa probably occurs due to environmental promoters in genetically susceptible tissues. For PCa, age and family history are predisposing factors and androgen is the promoter. Because the incidence of microscopic PCa appears independent of race and of geography despite very different incidence rates of clinically apparent disease, race may influence the progression of latent tumors to clinically evident tumors. Modest differences in androgen production among African-American, Asian and white men have been reported. These exposures over a lifetime may explain the influence of race on PCa.

The hereditary form is set apart from the more common form by an earlier age of onset. Hereditary PCa is rare, although positive family history confers significant risk for given individuals in that family.

Pathogenesis

Adenocarcinoma of the glandular epithelium of the peripheral zone of the prostate gland is the most common form of PCa. It results from androgen activity on a tissue with acquired oncogenic potential. **Prostatic intraepithelial neoplasia (PIN)** is the first sign of an evolving neoplastic process. It is characterized by proliferation and anaplasia of the cells lining the ducts and glandular acini of the **peripheral zone** and disruption of the architecture of the basal epithelial cell layers.

Like most malignancies, the prognosis in PCa is determined by the stage and grade of the tumor at detection. Patients with disease localized to the prostate have an 80% survival rate at 5 years. The presence of distant metastases at diagnosis significantly lowers 5-year survival. PCa spreads locally to the hypogastric and presacral chains of lymph nodes and hematogenously to bone.

The interaction between prostatic stroma and epithelium appears to have an important role in the development of PCa (Fig. 41.1b). Different stromal growth factors are overexpressed in PCa when compared with BPH. Specifically, the stroma of PCa contains more IGF, EGF and TGF-β, while that in BPH contains more bFGF. DHT and testosterone both stimulate production of EGF and TGF-β by the prostate gland. The androgen dependence of these growth factors probably also accounts for much of the hormonal dependence of the normal prostate gland.

Mutations in the *ERBB2* oncogene cause increased EGF receptor (EGFR) activity in PCa. Similar *ERBB2* mutations are found in breast cancers. In both diseases, the EGFR shifts from its normal position in the basal epithelial layer to the luminal epithelium as the disease progresses from hyperplasia to intraepithelial neoplasia to frank cancer. Hereditary PCa is associated with mutations in the *BRCA1* or *BRCA2* tumor suppressor genes. Similar gene mutations are also associated with breast and ovarian cancers.

Loss of heterogeneity studies have identified several chromosomal loci as potential sites for abnormal tumor suppressor activity in PCa. For instance, in PCa that metastasizes after therapy, there is a gain in genetic material at the site of the androgen receptor gene on the long arm of the X chromosome. The gene for the androgen receptor becomes amplified after androgen withdrawal treatment, an adaptation by the tumor that aids its survival under androgen-deficient conditions. This discovery sheds light on the molecular basis for the development of drug resistance by some cancer cells.

Prostate-specific antigen (PSA) is a protease secreted by the prostatic epithelium. Small amounts leak across the prostatic acini and into the plasma. PSA determinations may be used as a screening tool for PCa in asymptomatic men although the risk-benefit ratio of this approach remains unclear.

Treatment

Treatment of locally contained PCa includes surgery, radiation therapy or active surveillance. Surgical treatment involves removing the prostate and seminal vesicles in an effort to completely remove all malignant prostate cancer cells. With radiation therapy, radiation is delivered to the prostate either externally or internally with seeds placed inside prostate. Active surveillance (following the prostate cancer without specific treatment) may be used for those men who have small volume disease of the prostate or those who have significant comorbidities. In these patients, it is felt that the prostate cancer could grow slowly enough that treatment is not necessary. Other less common treatments for localized prostate cancer include cryosurgery (freezing of the prostate) and high-intensity focused ultrasound to the prostate.

Treatment of metastatic PCa involves androgen withdrawal, which may be accomplished by orchidectomy (surgical removal of the testicles), by treatment with leuteinizing hormone (LH) aka gonadotropin releasing hormone (GnRH) agonists or antagonists (both ultimatelysuppress LH release, or by treatment with an antiandrogen. Chemotherapy is used when hormonal withdrawal is not effective; it has modest success in treating metastatic PCa.

42 Ovarian neoplasms

The overwhelming majority of ovarian masses are benign and the lifetime risk of developing ovarian cancer is about 2%. Age is the most important factor in determining risk of malignancy. Adnexal masses are common during the reproductive years. During this stage of life, such masses are usually caused by functional ovarian cysts, benign neoplasms of the ovary or by postinfectious changes in the fallopian tubes. In girls under 20 and in women over 50, about 10% of all palpable ovarian masses are malignant. Between 85 and 90% of ovarian cancer occurs in postmenopausal women.

Benign neoplasms of the ovary

Benign and malignant neoplasms can develop from any cell type found in the ovary. Simple cysts can be functional and form at the site of ovulation or during the development of the corpus luteum. These are very common and distinguishable from true neoplasms by their transitory nature. They typically disappear within 6 weeks of discovery. Complex or solid masses and those that are persistent are more likely to be truly neoplastic and require histologic diagnosis.

Dermoids are a unique type of benign ovarian tumor that arises from more mature germ cells than the other germ-cell tumors (GCTs) found in women (Table 42.1). On gross examination, dermoids may contain hair, bone, cartilage and large amounts of greasy fluid that rapidly becomes sebaceous at room temperature. On histologic examination, the tumors contain disarrayed clusters of many of the cell types normally seen in fetuses. Like other GCTs, the molecular event(s) that lead to activation of the germ cells in dermoids can occur *in utero* and benign ovarian teratomas have been detected in the fetus and newborn infant. Ovarian dermoid tumors display abnormalities in imprinting and are discussed in more detail in Chapter 45.

Ovarian cancers

Ovarian cancer is the most lethal gynecologic malignancy. While over 90% of testicular malignancies are GCTs, 65–70% of ovarian malignancies are epithelial cell cancers. GCTs of the testis have good early detection and high cure rates (Chapter 40). Ovarian epithelial cell cancers are usually detected after widespread intraperitoneal dissemination. At this point, cure is almost impossible.

There are five distinct histologic types of epithelial ovarian tumors: **serous, mucinous, endometrioid, clear cell** and **Brenner**. Of the five, serous neoplasms account for almost half of all tumors. Mucinous tumors comprise about 25%, endometrioid tumors about 5%, clear cell cancers under 5% and Brenner cell tumors 2–3% of the total. The remainder of ovarian cancers are too poorly differentiated at diagnosis to be classified.

Epithelial ovarian cancer typically spreads both locally and by intraperitoneal dissemination. Contiguous spread is to the fallopian tube and uterus. Dissemination occurs to the contralateral ovary and peritoneum. Implants of epithelial ovarian cancer may be found on the cul-de-sac, bowel, mesentery, omentum and diaphragm. Malignant ascites forms when diaphragmatic metastases block the lymphatic drainage of the peritoneal cavity. Patients with these cancers may not develop symptoms until the tumor mass compresses other intraperitoneal organs or the associated ascites causes abdominal bloating, dyspepsia or urinary frequency. This relative lack of early symptoms leads

Table 42.1 Ovarian neoplasms

Ovarian neoplasms derived from epithelium
Serous tumor
Mucinous tumor
Endometrioid tumor
Mesonephroid (clear cell) tumor
Brenner tumor
Carcinosarcoma and mixed mesodermal tumor

Neoplasms derived from germ cells
Teratoma
    Mature teratoma
    Solid adult teratoma
    Dermoid cyst
    Struma ovarii (thyroid differentiation in >50% of mass)
    Malignant neoplasms secondarily arising from mature cystic
      teratoma
    Immature teratoma (partially differentiated teratoma)
Dysgerminoma
Embryonal carcinoma
Endodermal sinus tumor
Choriocarcinoma
Gonadoblastoma

Neoplasms derived from specialized gonadal stroma
Granulosa–theca cell tumor
    Granulosa tumor
    Thecoma
Sertoli–Leydig tumor
    Arrhenoblastoma
    Sertoli tumor
Gynandroblastoma
Lipid cell tumor

Neoplasms derived from nonspecific mesenchyme
Fibroma, hemangioma, leiomyoma, lipoma
Lymphoma
Sarcoma

Neoplasms metastatic to the ovary
Gastrointestinal tract (Krukenberg)
Breast
Endometrium
Lymphoma

to late diagnosis and poor prognosis. Treatment for epithelial ovarian cancer involves cytoreductive surgery and aggressive chemotherapy, and only 15% of patients with advanced disease will survive. These tumors often develop resistance to chemotherapy. When disease is confined to the ovary, survival dramatically improves to 50–90%. Unfortunately, ovarian epithelial tumors are seldom diagnosed at this early stage.

About 15% of all epithelial ovarian cancers have histologic and biologic behaviors that are neither clearly benign nor frankly malignant. These "borderline" ovarian carcinomas share a common genetic lineage with their corresponding benign cystic neoplasms. Borderline tumors have a 95% 10-year survival rate but can recur as many as 20 years after excision. Late recurrences are often identical to the primary

The Reproductive System at a Glance, Fourth Edition. Linda J. Heffner and Danny J. Schust.

tumor, but malignant transformation to high-grade epithelial ovarian cancer can occur in a minority of cases.

Epidemiology of epithelial ovarian cancer

Family history is the most important risk factor, followed by age. The mean age of disease onset is 59 years. Other risk factors are early menarche, late menopause, regular and uninterrupted menstrual cycles, short menstrual cycle length, low parity and a history of infertility. High parity and use of oral contraceptives reduce the risk of ovarian cancer. Both also decrease the number of lifetime ovulation events. These epidemiologic data suggest that the number of ovulations over a lifetime is significant in the pathogenesis of the disease.

As with other prevalent epithelial cancers, environmental factors influence the development of ovarian cancers, with the highest rates being found in highly industrialized countries. Japan is the single notable exception, with rates of malignant neoplasms of the ovary that are among the lowest in the world. However, the rates in Japanese immigrants in the USA approach those of Caucasian natives within two to three generations, suggesting that carcinogens in the immediate environment are responsible. Chemical carcinogens from the outside world can reach the pelvic peritoneum of women through the vagina and upper reproductive tract. In fact, investigators have shown that more women with ovarian cancer use talc as a dusting powder on their perineum or sanitary napkins than matched controls. The association between talc and ovarian cancer is also biologically plausible. Talc is chemically related to asbestos and ovarian cancer is similar to the mesotheliomas that can develop after pulmonary exposure to asbestos.

Familial ovarian cancer

Various syndromes have been have been associated with increased risk for the development of cancers. Three include a predisposition to ovarian cancer: familial ovarian cancer syndrome, hereditary breast/ovarian cancer syndrome and Lynch cancer family syndrome II (hereditary nonpolyposis colorectal cancer syndrome, HNPCC). These syndromes account for less than 10% of ovarian cancer diagnoses. Virtually all the hereditary breast/ovarian cancers and site-specific ovarian cancer syndromes are caused by mutations in the tumor suppressor genes *BRCA1* or *BRCA2*. Individuals with *BRCA1* mutations have a 20-fold increase in their risk for developing both breast and ovarian cancers, and those with *BRCA2* mutations a 5–10-fold increase in their risk for developing ovarian cancer. The estimated frequency of *BRCA1* mutations in the general population is 1 in 800, but is greater than 1 in 100 among Ashkenazi Jewish women. *BRCA2* mutations have a very similar carrier frequency among the Ashkenazi and a frequency of 1 in 250 among Icelanders.

HNPCC is caused by mutations in any one of several genes important in DNA mismatch repair. The most common extracolonic malignancy in women with HNPCC is endometrial cancer, followed by ovarian cancer.

Pathogenesis of nonfamilial epithelial ovarian cancer

The typical advanced stage of epithelial ovarian cancers at clinical presentation, combined with the lack of identifiable precursor lesions for the more common serous and mucinous adenocarcinomas, have made biologic study of their development difficult. Originally, some investigators proposed that epithelial ovarian cancers arise in small inclusion cysts that develop when surface epithelial cells become entrapped in the physical defects left in the ovarian surface after ovulation while others hypothesized that the ovarian epithelium is a coelomic mesothelium that is more prone to metaplasia than other epithelia. More recent studies suggest that many ovarian tumors may actually originate in other pelvic organs and involve the ovary secondarily. Serous tumors may arise from fallopian tube epithelium that either implants or is trapped in the ovary at the time of ovulatory capsule disruption. Endometrioid and clear cell tumors, both of which are associated with the clinical condition of endometriosis (Chapter 34), may arise when endometrium menstruates retrograde onto the ovary although coelomic metaplasia may also be involved. Metaplasia of tissue at the tubal mesothelial junction may give rise to mucinous and Brenner tumors. It has been argued by some that ovarian malignancies are more appropriately classified into two groups of tumors based both on morphology and molecular genetic features. When this is done, the members of one group each share lineage with a paired benign neoplasm and behave rather indolently while the other group frequently displays tumor suppressor abnormalities that involve p53, the product of a tumor suppressing cell checkpoint gene located on chromosome 17p, and progress rapidly. The first group is comprised low-grade serous, low-grade endometrioid, clear cell, mucinous and transitional (Brenner) tumors. Each histologic group exhibits a distinctive molecular genetic profile and all lack p53 mutations. The second group includes high-grade serous carcinoma, undifferentiated carcinomas and mixed mesodermal tumors (carcinosarcoma).

As with other malignancies, ovarian cancer probably develops after multiple genetic "hits" cause a cell to display invasive, neoplastic behavior. One "hit" typically involves activation of an oncogene and the second "hit" involves the loss of one or more genes with tumor suppressor activity. *BRCA1* and *BRCA2* are tumor suppressor genes and inheritance of one abnormal allele makes "second hits" a high statistical probability.

Other ovarian malignancies

Only 10% of ovarian cancers are GCTs. These occur largely in girls and young women. Like GCTs in men, GCTs in women arise from immature germ cells and include five distinct histologic types: **dysgerminomas**, **choriocarcinomas**, **endodermal sinus tumors** (yolk sac carcinomas), **embryonal carcinomas** and **teratomas**. The dysgerminoma is the female equivalent of the seminoma. GCTs of the testes are typically detected early in their development; GCTs of the ovary are not. For this reason, far less is known about GCT tumorigenesis in the female than in the male (Chapter 40).

Stromal cell tumors are the rarest ovarian malignancies, accounting for 5% of the total. They may contain granulosa, theca, Leydig or Sertoli cells, and usually make large amounts of steroid hormones: granulosa or theca cell tumors make estrogens and Leydig or Sertoli cell tumors make androgens. The occurrence of stromal cell tumors is not age dependent. Those secreting androgens can cause virilization while those secreting estrogens can cause endometrial hyperplasia and irregular vaginal bleeding.

Carcinoma of the uterine endometrium is the most common pelvic malignancy in women. The USA and Canada have the highest incidence rates in the world, whereas developing countries and Japan have incidence rates four to five times lower. Epidemiologic data indicate that there are two forms of endometrial cancer. One is directly related to estrogen exposure and is most common in the USA. The other is unrelated to estrogen and occurs throughout the world. Estrogen-related type I tumors occur among younger perimenopausal women and carry a good prognosis. In fact, type I lesions are potentially preventable through recognition of patient risk, diagnosis of the precursor lesion (atypical endometrial hyperplasia) and proper treatment. Non-estrogen-related type II tumors occur in older postmenopausal women without a history of estrogen exposure and have a poorer prognosis. The molecular genetic alterations present in type I and II endometrial carcinomas are distinct and may help to explain their clinical characteristics.

Cells of the Müllerian tract can differentiate into a wide range of tissue types. This is demonstrated by the variety of histologic subtypes seen among the endometrial cancers. The vast majority are endometrioid adenocarcinomas. Prognosis for patients with endometrioid adenocarcinoma is determined largely by its degree of differentiation or histologic grade (well, moderately or poorly differentiated). In fact, histologic grade is a prognostic factor independent of stage at diagnosis. Less common histologic subtypes include mucinous adenocarcinoma, serous adenocarcinoma, clear cell adenocarcinoma, squamous cell carcinoma and a variety of rare mixed and undifferentiated tumors. For all subtypes other than endometrioid adenocarcinoma, prognosis depends more on histologic subtype than on histologic grade.

Endometrioid adenocarcinoma first invades the stroma of the underlying uterine tissue by destroying the glandular basement membrane. It then invades the myometrium and cervix. Endometrioid adenocarcinoma typically spreads via the pelvic and periaortic lymphatic channels rather than hematogenously. Vascular invasion is usually seen only with high-grade, non-estrogen-dependent lesions.

Treatment of endometrial cancer usually involves surgical removal of the uterus, fallopian tubes and ovaries. Patients with deep myometrial invasion or disease outside of the uterus may be treated postoperatively with radiation, chemotherapy or progestin-based hormonal therapies. Pretreatment analysis of endometrioid adenocarcinoma specimens for estrogen and progesterone receptor status may help to direct postsurgical therapy. There is a good correlation between tumor differentiation and receptor content. Well-differentiated tumors usually have greater numbers of estrogen and progesterone receptors. Because receptor content predicts response to progestin therapy, patients with well-differentiated tumors may be good candidates for progestin therapy.

The survival rate for endometrial cancer is relatively good. Overall, survival approaches 70% at both 5 and 10 years. Patients with stage 1 disease, in which the tumor has not invaded through more than half the myometrial thickness, have a 5-year survival rate of over 90%. Because of its high prevalence, endometrial cancer can be considered a neoplasia of high morbidity and relatively low mortality in developed countries.

Epidemiology of endometrial cancer

Endometrial cancer is largely a disease of the postmenopausal woman. About 80% of cases diagnosed are in women aged 50–75 years of age,

Table 43.1 Risk factors for endometrial cancer

Increased risk
Obesity
Diabetes
High-fat diet
High socioeconomic status
Urban residence
Positive family history
Polycystic ovary syndrome
Unopposed estrogen replacement therapy in menopause
Tamoxifen use
Estrogen-secreting tumors

Decreased risk
Delayed menarche
Combination oral contraceptive use
Child-bearing

with peak incidence in those aged 55–70. A woman entering menopause has double the chance of developing endometrial cancer compared with her chance for developing carcinoma of the cervix or the ovary. The incidence of endometrial cancer varies dramatically from country to country. This geographic pattern follows that of breast and ovarian cancer, with the highest rates in industrialized countries. It is exactly the opposite of patterns observed for cervical cancer.

An association between estrogen exposure and endometrial cancer has been apparent for over 50 years. Many of the risk factors listed in Table 43.1 are thought to increase the risk because of their close association with high estrogen levels, typically unopposed by progesterone. The single most important and best defined risk factor for adenocarcinoma of the uterus is obesity. Adipose tissue has active aromatase enzymes. Adrenal androgens are rapidly converted to estrogens within the adipose tissue of obese individuals. These newly synthesized estrogens also have excellent bioavailability because the metabolic changes associated with obesity inhibit the production of sex hormone-binding globulins by the liver. Obese individuals may have dramatic elevations in their circulating bioavailable estrogens and this exposure can cause hyperplastic growth of the endometrium.

Close links exist between the risk of endometrial cancer, a high-fat diet and gross national product, which suggests that level of industrial development may affect incidence of endometrial carcinoma by influencing food consumption. A high-fat diet is also associated with obesity and type 2 diabetes mellitus. Amount and type of dietary fat influences estrogen metabolism. For example, diets rich in beef or in fats increase estrogen reabsorption from the bowel.

White women are three times more likely to be diagnosed with endometrial cancer than black women. Again, this is exactly the opposite of what is seen for cervical cancer.

Steroid hormones and endometrial cancer

As noted above, the epidemiologic data on endometrial cancer reveal a striking association between estrogen exposure and cancer develop-

The Reproductive System at a Glance, Fourth Edition. Linda J. Heffner and Danny J. Schust.

94 © 2014 John Wiley & Sons, Ltd. Published 2014 by John Wiley & Sons, Ltd. Companion Website: www.ataglanceseries.com/reproduction

ment. Interestingly, a direct causal link can only be inferred at this time. The basis for considering estrogen as an etiologic factor comes from three sources: (i) the biologic activity of estrogen and progesterone on the endometrium; (ii) animal and human data on the effects of diethylstilbestrol (DES) on carcinogenesis; and (iii) the association of endometrial cancer with endometrial hyperplasia in conjunction with the association of hyperplasia with prolonged and unopposed estrogen exposure.

The strongest attestation to the high sensitivity of the endometrium to ovarian steroid hormones is the dramatic changes that occur in this tissue during each menstrual cycle (Chapters 10 and 14). In a normally cycling woman, the endometrium changes its morphology on a day-to-day basis. In the follicular phase of the cycle, estrogens stimulate proliferation of the epithelium covering the endometrial glands and of the underlying stroma. Estrogen induces production of its own receptor and of the progesterone receptor during this time. Progesterone secreted after ovulation promptly arrests the proliferative activity in the glands and converts the epithelium to a secretory state. The stroma responds to progesterone with angiogenesis and functional maturation. If pregnancy should occur, these changes will prepare the endometrium for implantation. It is believed that the potent mitogenic effect of estrogen on the epithelium of the endometrial glands accelerates the spontaneous mutation rate of predisposing oncogenes and/or tumor suppressor genes. This leads to neoplastic transformation.

Animal and human data gathered after developmental exposure to DES add biologic evidence for the carcinogenic potential of estrogens in the reproductive tract. DES is a nonsteroidal estrogen agonist that was among the first synthetic estrogens to be developed. It was administered to over 2 million women between 1940 and 1970 as treatment for threatened miscarriage. In mice, neonatal exposure to DES produces endometrial cancer in 95% of animals by 18 months of age. In women, prenatal DES exposure leads to structural abnormalities of the reproductive tract (Chapter 27) and to clear cell adenocarcinoma of the vagina and cervix. The carcinogenic action of the DES appears to be mediated in part through activation of the estrogen receptor. Whether prenatal DES exposure will cause endometrial cancer in humans will be determined as this cohort of women continues to be followed through menopause. The molecular genetic mechanism by which DES lead to clear cell carcinoma and naturally occurring estrogens to type I endometrial cancer may be similar. Genetic instability of microsatellite sequences has been demonstrated in both of these tumors.

Molecular biology of endometrial cancer

K-*ras* oncogene mutations and microsatellite instability are most common in type I estrogen-related tumors. Mutations of the *PT53* tumor suppressor gene and overexpression of the *ERBB2* oncogene are more frequently observed in type II non-estrogen-related tumors.

Endometrial hyperplasia

Endometrial hyperplasia describes a spectrum of changes in the endometrium. These can range from slightly disordered patterns that merely exaggerate the changes seen in the late proliferative stage of the menstrual cycle to irregular, hyperchromatic lesions that are difficult to distinguish from endometrioid adenocarcinoma. Nonetheless, noninvasive endometrial hyperplasia can be divided into two basic types: hyperplasia and atypical hyperplasia. Atypia is characterized by nuclear enlargement, hyperchromasia or irregularities in nuclear shape. Hyperplastic lesions can be further subdivided. Simple hyperplasia describes hyperplastic changes with regular glandular architecture while complex hyperplasia has irregular glandular architecture (Fig. 43.1a). Of the four types of endometrial hyperplasias – simple, complex, atypical simple and atypical complex – only atypical complex hyperplasia poses significant risk for progression to invasive carcinoma. The progression from hyperplasia is slow and may take 5 years or more. About 20% of women with complex atypical hyperplasia will develop endometrial adenocarcinoma (Fig. 43.1b). Only 1–2% of those with the other hyperplastic lesions will progress.

Endometrial hyperplasia has the same epidemiologic risk factors as endometrial cancer. Among patients with atypical endometrial hyperplasia, postmenopausal status is associated with the highest risk of progression to adenocarcinoma (33% over 10 years). Endometrial cancer is rare during the child-bearing years. When it occurs, it is usually associated with clinical disorders that cause chronic, unopposed estrogen exposure, including the polycystic ovary syndrome and chronic anovulation (Chapter 31). Estrogen-producing ovarian tumors, such as the granulosa–theca cell tumors (Chapter 42), are also associated with the development of endometrial hyperplasia and adenocarcinoma in premenopausal women.

Progesterone-based therapies are used to halt endometrial proliferation and to convert the endometrium to a secretory state in women with endometrial hyperplasia with low malignant potential. Treatment can be given cyclically or continuously. Atypical endometrial hyperplasia is treated surgically (hysterectomy) unless there is a contraindication to the procedure.

Figure 43.1 (a) Simple endometrial hyperplasia

Figure 43.1 (b) Well-differentiated endometrial adenocarcinoma

44 Cervical cancer

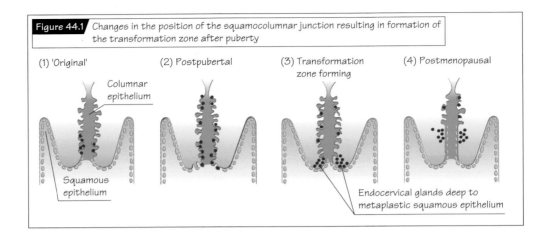

Figure 44.1 Changes in the position of the squamocolumnar junction resulting in formation of the transformation zone after puberty

(1) 'Original'

Columnar epithelium

Squamous epithelium

(2) Postpubertal

(3) Transformation zone forming

Endocervical glands deep to metaplastic squamous epithelium

(4) Postmenopausal

Invasive squamous cell carcinoma accounts for 80% of cervical malignancies. Unlike the remainder of the reproductive tract cancers, which are more prevalent in industrialized countries, cervical cancer ranks second in cancer mortality in developing nations. Virtually all cervical cancers are associated with the human papillomavirus (HPV), which is the most common sexually transmitted infection. Squamous cancer of the cervix is unique in that it is a preventable disease when vaccination, proper screening and treatment are available and employed.

Like prostatic cancer in men (Chapter 41), cervical cancer typically arises from a precursor lesion, cervical intraepithelial neoplasia (CIN). CIN is asymptomatic and appears to precede invasive carcinoma of the cervix by 5–15 years. Almost all cervical cancer arises in the transformation zone (squamocolumnar junction) of the cervix. Here, the columnar, glandular epithelium of the endocervix meets the squamous epithelium of the ectocervix. The anatomic location of the squamocolumnar junction changes in response to a variety of factors and is different in young postpubertal girls when compared with postmenopausal women (Fig. 44.1). In older women, the transformation zone may be high in the endocervical canal. This makes the early diagnosis of cervical neoplasia more difficult.

Cervical carcinomas can spread in any one of four ways: (i) directly into the vaginal mucosa; (ii) directly into the myometrium of the lower uterine segment; (iii) into the paracervical lymphatics and from there to the obturator, hypogastric and external iliac lymph nodes; and (iv) directly into adjacent structures such as the bladder anteriorly, the rectum posteriorly, or the parametrial tissues and pelvic sidewalls laterally. Lymphatic invasion can occur even when cervical tumors are still small. Hematogenous spread and distant metastases are usually very late manifestations of the disease.

Surgical treatment is used for early-stage cervical cancers. A combination of radiation and chemotherapy is used for patients with advanced disease and in those who are poor surgical candidates.

Epidemiology of cervical cancer

The association of sexual activity with cervical cancer was first identified over 150 years ago when it was noted that the disease was rare in nuns and frequent in prostitutes. Subsequent epidemiologic data have identified the onset of sexual activity in adolescence and multiple sexual partners as high-risk characteristics for cervical cancer. Its incidence is higher in low-income women but this effect is not independent of early sexual activity and multiple sex partners. Smoking is an independent risk factor for the development of cervical cancer. Characteristics of a "high-risk" male partner include men whose previous partner developed cervical cancer, who themselves develop penile cancer or who have not had a circumcision.

Epidemiologic data suggesting that cervical cancer behaves like a sexually transmitted disease led to identification of HPV as the causative agent. Although it has been identified in over 99% of all cervical cancers, HPV infection of the cervix appears necessary but not sufficient for the development of cervical cancer. This distinction is important as cervical infection with HPV is very common; however, the majority of these infections are transient. Persistent infection with an oncogenic type of HPV confers an increased risk of developing cervical cancer.

Pathogenesis of squamous cell neoplasia of the cervix

Because the cervix is so physically accessible, the pathogenesis of cervical neoplasia has been studied extensively. Pathogenesis clearly involves exposure of a vulnerable tissue (the transformation zone) to carcinogens.

The squamocolumnar junction is one of six epithelial boundaries present within the lower genital tract. The position of the squamocolumnar junction is affected by the hormonal and anatomical changes of puberty, pregnancy and menopause (Fig. 44.1). Prior to puberty, the squamocolumnar junction is at the level of the external cervical os (Chapter 9). With puberty, estrogen-induced changes in the shape and volume of the cervix carry the squamocolumnar junction out onto the anatomic ectocervix. This repositioning exposes tissues previously found in the lower endocervical canal to the vaginal environment. The exposure of the simple mucin-secreting epithelium to the acidic vaginal milieu induces a chemical denaturation of the villus tips of the columnar epithelium. The reparative process that follows eventually produces a mature squamous epithelium. **After menopause, the**

The Reproductive System at a Glance, Fourth Edition. Linda J. Heffner and Danny J. Schust.

squamocolumnar junction retreats to a position high within the endocervical canal.

HPV is a DNA virus that causes epithelial lesions in the skin, cervix, vagina, vulva (Chapter 47), anus and oropharynx. More than 100 types of HPV have been identified to date. The HPV infections affecting the genital tract are classified according to their oncogenic potential. The highest risk HPV genotypes are 16 and 18, which have been detected in 65% of cervical cancers.

Cervical infection with HPV is very common – 80% of all sexually active women will have at least one infection with HPV; however, the majority of these infections are transient. The average duration of infection is 8 months, and 90% of HPV infections in young women will clear within 2 years. It is thought that the local immune response of the host is primarily responsible for HPV clearance; only persistent (greater than 6–12 months' duration) HPV infection puts the cervix at risk for changes that could develop into cancer. **Typically, HPV infection persists for greater than 10 years before causing carcinogenesis.** Women with an impaired immune system, such as HIV-infected women, have high rates of persistent cervical HPV infections and cervical neoplasia.

Cervical intraepithelial neoplasia (CIN) is the term used to encompass all premalignant epithelial abnormalities of the cervix. It has replaced an older terminology that used the terms "dysplasia" and "carcinoma *in situ*" of the cervix. **CIN, although divided into grades, is actually a single neoplastic continuum.** The designations CIN1, 2 and 3 reflect the extent of the cellular aberrations within the cervical

epithelium (Fig. 44.2). For instance, in CIN1, the lower one-third of the epithelial cells (closest to the basement membrane) lack evidence of differentiation or maturation. This exit from the normal differentiation pathway signals neoplastic transformation.

Screening tests for cervical cancer

The cervical smear or **Pap test** (named after Dr. George Papanicolaou who developed the test) was designed as a screening test to detect squamous cell abnormalities. Its success is based on the fact that the nuclear abnormalities of neoplastic cervical cells are present in samples that are scraped or exfoliated from the surface of the cervix. In countries where cervical cancer screening with Pap testing is routinely performed, the incidence and mortality rates of cervical cancer have both decreased by 70%. It is likely that the treatment of premalignant lesions and the finding of earlier stage cervical cancers have contributed to the decreased incidence and mortality of cervical cancer.

HPV tests of the cervix can be used as an adjunct to cervical cytology screening for women aged 30 years and over. HPV testing for primary screening of younger women is not recommended because of the high rates of transient HPV infections that would be detected. The benefits of adding HPV testing include: (i) a reliable, readily reproducible measure of the risk of disease; (ii) a high negative predictive value with a single test that allows prolongation of the screening interval; and (iii) increased sensitivity (although lower specificity) compared with cervical cytology in the detection of CIN2–3.

Prophylactic HPV vaccination

Two prophylactic HPV vaccines based on virus-like particles (VLPs) have been developed. Both provide protection against HPV types 16 and 18 – the causative agent for approximately 65% of cervical cancers worldwide. HPV vaccines prevent the development of HPV 16 and 18 infections, HPV 16 and 18 associated CIN2 or 3, adenocarcinoma *in situ* and invasive cervical cancer, with 98% efficacy in young women without prior HPV 16 or 18 infection. Vaccination is recommended for girls who are not yet sexually active as HPV infections rates are very high among adolescents. Interestingly, the mechanism of action of these vaccines is not well understood as the primary mode of natural immunity to HPV is a local immune response and not a systemic response.

Cervical adenocarcinoma

Adenocarcinoma of the cervix is much rarer than squamous cell lesions. It occurs most often in women during the reproductive years and is frequently associated with HPV type 16 or 18. Although adenocarcinoma *in situ* is thought to be the precursor lesion of invasive cervical adenocarcinoma, the timing of progression from precursor to invasion is not well-defined. Cervical cytology does not reliably detect adenocarcinomas but may detect concomitantly present cervical squamous neoplasia; HPV testing should have improved sensitivity for the detection of adenocarcinomas.

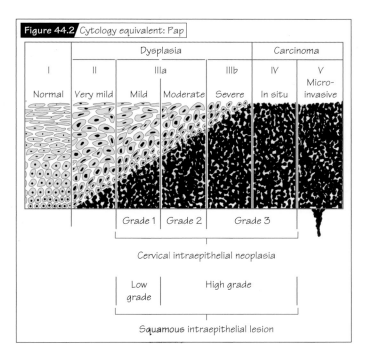

Figure 44.2 Cytology equivalent: Pap

Genetic imprinting and reproductive tract tumors

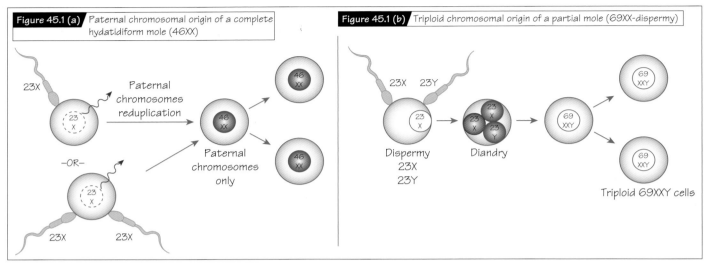

Figure 45.1 (a) Paternal chromosomal origin of a complete hydatidiform mole (46XX)

Figure 45.1 (b) Triploid chromosomal origin of a partial mole (69XX-dispermy)

Imprinting

Imprinting is the differential expression of a gene or set of genes that is determined by whether that genetic material was inherited from the mother or from the father. During the imprinting process, specific genes are methylated so that they can no longer be transcribed. Therefore, for certain genetic loci, only the information from one parent is transcriptionally active. When a gene is maternally imprinted, the gene acquired from the mother is inactive and that from the father is transcribed. With paternal imprinting, the allele acquired from the father is inactive. Normal embryonic development requires that one set of genes be maternally imprinted and a second paternally imprinted. Therefore, a zygote must not only have a 2*n* chromosome content but each of the 1*n* components must derive from different parents. Several tumors of the reproductive system have helped us to better understand the process of imprinting and the consequences of imprinting abnormalities.

Gestational trophoblastic disease (GTD), dermoid cysts of the ovary and germ-cell tumors (GCTs) of the testis all display abnormalities in imprinting. GTD and dermoid tumors contain two sets of chromosomes from a single parent, so there exists no opportunity for biparental imprinting. Two sets of maternally imprinted genes are present in dermoid tumors of the ovary. The result is development of disorganized fetal tissues without any supporting placenta or fetal membranes. Conversely, two sets of paternally imprinted genes are present in GTD. In these cases, dysplastic trophoblast develops, but a fetus does not. GCTs of the testis have taught different lessons concerning the importance of imprinting. GCTs that arise in immature and incompletely imprinted cells are more aggressive than those that arise in fully imprinted germ cells.

Gestational trophoblastic disease

GTD is one of the earliest reported neoplasms. Hippocrates first described "dropsy" of the uterus in 400 BC and a 13th century tombstone noted the birth of 365 "children," half boys and half girls, to the woman buried there. Today GTD, also called molar pregnancy, retains its leading position in tumor biology as the most sensitive and curable of all human cancers. The genetic origin of molar pregnancies has also played a pivotal part in our understanding of the role of the maternal and paternal genome in embryonic development.

There is a spectrum of diseases within the GTD classification: hydatidiform mole, either complete (CHM) or partial (PHM), persistent, nonmetastatic GTD, metastatic good-prognosis GTD and metastatic poor-prognosis GTD. The latter includes aggressive tumors known as choriocarcinomas (CC). Of these, CHM and PHM follow abnormal conceptions and are restricted to women. CC is unique among GTD in that it can arise from a normal conception, a molar pregnancy or a germ-cell line. CC in men is exclusively of germ-cell origin (Chapter 40).

CHM and PHM contain two sets of paternal chromosomes (Fig. 45.1). The former has only paternally derived genomic DNA. This situation promotes the development of placental tissues in the absence of fetal tissue development. In PHM, two sets of paternal chromosomes are accompanied by a single set of maternal chromosomes. Again, the paternally imprinted genes are duplicated and placental overgrowth occurs. Here, maternally imprinted genes are also present and fetal tissue development is seen.

Complete hydatidiform mole

CHM is the most common of the GTDs and occurs in about 1 in 1000–1500 pregnancies in Western countries. It is at least twice as common in Asia but less common in black races. Extremes of age increase the risk for CHM, with women under 15 and over 40 at highest risk. Other risk factors include previous history of CHM, previous miscarriage, maternal balanced chromosomal translocation, professional occupation and perhaps deficiencies in animal fat and carotene in the diet. A previously normal pregnancy lowers the risk of CHM.

CHM is characterized histologically by the presence of large amounts of hydropic placental villi and no fetal tissue. It presents clinically with delayed menses and the diagnosis of pregnancy. Pregnancy symptoms such as nausea and vomiting are often exaggerated because of the high human chorionic gonadotropin (hCG) production by the abnormal trophoblast. Some patients with CHM will be hyperthyroid because hCG exhibits some intrinsic thyroid-stimulating activity.

Women with CHM who want to preserve their fertility are treated by removing the molar tissue from the uterine cavity (uterine evacuation). Those who do not desire future fertility may choose hysterectomy. Eighty per cent of CHMs will respond to these approaches. Those who

The Reproductive System at a Glance, Fourth Edition. Linda J. Heffner and Danny J. Schust.

Figure 45.2 An ovarian dermoid tumor can contain an array of cell types

Hair

Sebaceous gland

Squamous epithelia

have persistent disease require chemotherapy and the vast majority will ultimately be cured. CHM is exquisitely sensitive to antimetabolite chemotherapy, typically methotrexate with folate rescue.

The unique genetic origins of CHM were suspected well before the advent of modern molecular techniques when karyotype analyses revealed that 96% of them were 46XX. Polymerase chain reaction and restriction fragment length polymorphism (RFLP) analyses have demonstrated that **while CHM is always diploid, the chromosomes are all of paternal origin**. Most CHMs arise from fertilization of an enucleate, or empty egg, with a single 23X sperm. This paternal haplotype reduplicates and the 46XX karyotype results. The remaining CHMs arise after fertilization of the enucleate egg with two sperm (dispermy); of these about one-quarter (4% of the total CHMs) will have a 46XY karyotype. All CHM have maternal mitochondrial DNA and this confirms that the oocyte cell machinery is involved. To date, the mechanism by which the egg enucleates is not known. Some hypothesize that the maternal chromosomes degenerate, others pose that the female pronucleus is extruded with the polar body (Chapters 4 and 16).

Partial hydatidiform mole

PHM exists when proliferative villi with hydropic degeneration coexist with a fetus. The fetus is genetically abnormal and will commonly die by the late first or early second trimester. The villous hydropic changes seen in PHM are not as pronounced as those in CHM and may be missed on ultrasonographic examination. Pathologic examination of the placenta is often necessary to make the diagnosis. Patients with PHM tend to be older than those with CHM. PHM has a lower risk of subsequent malignancy than does CHM.

PHM pregnancies are all triploid and contain two copies of the paternal genome. PHM pregnancies most commonly arise from dispermic fertilization (diandry). They occasionally occur after fertilization by a diploid sperm that failed to undergo a first or second reduction division during meiosis (Chapter 4).

Persistent and metastatic gestational trophoblastic disease

Persistent and metastatic GTD are typically preceded by CHM. They occasionally follow PHM or even normal pregnancies. Persistent GTD can invade the uterus or metastasize to liver, lung and brain. Even metastatic disease has a very high cure rate with appropriate treatment.

Genetic study of neoplastic trophoblastic tissue is very important to the patient because gestational tumors have a better than 90% cure rate whereas nongestational tumors with trophoblastic differentiation are essentially lethal.

Dermoid tumors

Benign ovarian teratomas, also known as **dermoids**, arise from "parthenogenetic" activation of premeiotic oocytes. Parthenogenetic activation of the oocyte stimulates oocyte mitosis in the absence of the male pronucleus and its accompanying DNA. Parthenogenetic activation can be induced *in vitro* by a variety of methods, including chemical and electrical exposure. The stimuli that drive parthenogenesis in the formation of ovarian teratomas are not known. All the chromosomes in an ovarian dermoid tumor are maternally derived and, therefore, maternally imprinted. The tumors are characterized by disorganized overgrowth of many of the cell types normally seen in fetuses. This includes hair, bone, cartilage, adipose tissue and glandular derivatives (Fig. 45.2).

Ovarian dermoid tumors arise from more mature germ cells than the other female GCTs (Chapter 42). Like other GCTs, the molecular event(s) that lead to activation of the germ cells can occur *in utero*, and indeed dermoid tumors have been detected in the fetus and newborn infant.

GCTs of the testis

Spermatocytic seminomas are unique among the GCTs of the testis in that they are found in older men and are typically slow-growing (Chapter 40). This less aggressive behavior may occur because spermatocytic seminomas arise from mature spermatogonia rather than spermatogonial stem cells. During the development of spermatozoa, the diploid (biparental) spermatogonial stem cell must undergo reduction division to the haploid state. It is equally important that the DNA in these haploid cells be completely uniparental. If this occurs, appropriate paternally imprinted DNA will be transmitted during fertilization. Imprinting appears to occur during spermatocyte maturation some time after the second meiotic division halves the chromosome number. When neoplastic transformation occurs in immature testicular germ cells, the biparental imprinting of the cells preserves pluripotentiality and allows the development of less differentiated, aggressive tumors with embryonal or trophoblastic components. When transformation occurs in more mature and fully imprinted spermatogonium, the tumors are less aggressive (spermatocytic seminomas).

Figure 46.1 Events observed during interaction between fallopian tube and N. gonorrhoeae gonococci (GC)

(1) Attachment of GC by pili to non-ciliated epithelial cells.

(2) Endocytosis of GC by cell and LPS mediated cytotoxic effects on adjacent cells.

(3) Movement of endocytoxic vacuole through cell to subepithelial space.

(4) Release of GC into subepithelial space.

Gonorrhea

Gonorrhea is the most frequently reported communicable disease in many of the more developed countries. Rates are 5–50 times higher than in the less developed world. The Gram-negative coccus that causes the disease is called *Neisseria gonorrhoeae*. It is a highly specialized organism that requires a mucosal surface to gain access to the body. **The most important health consequence of gonorrheal infections is fallopian tube damage and the associated predisposition to ectopic (tubal) pregnancies and infertility**.

In men, urethritis is the most common clinical manifestation of gonorrhea. Symptoms include dysuria and/or a purulent urethral discharge. Complications of gonorrhea are uncommon in men, but urethral stricture, epididymitis and prostatitis can occur. Between 20 and 30% of heterosexual men with symptomatic gonococcal urethritis are simultaneously infected with *Chlamydia trachomatis*.

Gonococcal infection in women is often asymptomatic. Morbidity associated with the infection, however, is far greater than that seen among infected men. A significant number of women diagnosed with gonorrhea are identified in sexually transmitted disease (STD) clinics as the asymptomatic consort of an infected partner. Uncomplicated urogenital gonococcal infection in women may present as dysuria from urethritis, vaginal discharge from cervicitis, or purulent drainage from the Skene or Bartholin glands at the vaginal introitus. **Pelvic inflammatory disease (PID)** is a term used to describe infection of the upper genital tract, including endometritis, salpingitis and peritonitis. *Neisseria gonorrhoeae* and *C. trachomatis* are the two pathogens most commonly isolated from women with positive cultures for PID. Women with **gonococcal PID** present with lower abdominal pain, abnormal uterine bleeding, dyspareunia (pain with intercourse) and fever. Although mortality from PID is low, morbidity is extremely high. PID is an important risk factor for chronic pelvic pain, infertility and tubal pregnancies. In some areas of Africa, up to 50% of women are infertile as a result of tubal occlusion from gonococcal PID.

Other serious clinical manifestations include disseminated gonococcal infection (DGI) and gonococcal ophthalmia neonatorum, a severe form of conjunctivitis affecting newborn infants who acquire the infection in the birth canal. Neonatal gonococcal ophthalmia can result in blindness if left untreated. It is a rarity in developed countries because neonatal ocular prophylaxis is mandated at birth, but remains a significant problem in many resource-poor parts of the world.

Gonorrhea is treated with antibiotics. Due to antibiotic resistence profiles, a parenteral cephalosporin plus doxycycline or azithromycin is currently first-line therapy for uncomplicated infections, but the choice of antibiotic evolves with resistence profiles and the propensity for the organism to be associated with other STDs.

Epidemiology of gonorrhea

Gonorrhea is largely a disease of youth. Incidence peaks in men and women at ages 18–24 years. In addition to age, the risk factors include low socioeconomic status, urban residence, unmarried status, non-white race, male homosexuality and prostitution.

Biology of *N. gonorrhoeae*

Gonococci enter the body by attaching to nonciliated columnar mucosal epithelial cells using specialized surface structures on the bacteria known as **pili** (Fig. 46.1). Following attachment by the pili, the gonococci are endocytosed by the cell. At this stage, a lipopolysaccharide (LPS; endotoxin)-mediated event is activated and nearby cells are killed. Following endocytosis of the bacteria, vacuoles containing viable and replicating gonococci pass through the cell from the mucosal surface to the subepithelial membrane. They are then released into the underlying tissues. The surface damage caused by the gonococcus allows other pathogens, such as chlamydia, to gain access to the upper reproductive tract and cause multiorganism PID. Movement of the gonococci to subepithelial sites also explains frequent failure to document its presence in the fallopian tube despite cervical culture-positive PID.

Gonococci develop their antibiotic resistance through plasmid-mediated and chromosomal mechanisms. Most plasmid-mediated resistance is to penicillin and tetracycline. Chromosomally mediated resistance is more general and involves mutations that alter cell wall permeability or the affinity of binding proteins to antibiotics.

Chlamydia

There are many similarities between the infections caused by *N. gonorrhoeae* and **Chlamydia trachomatis (CT)**. Chlamydiae access the body by invading the same epithelial cells of the endocervix, urethra, endometrium, fallopian tubes, rectum and conjunctivae that are host to the gonococcus. Infections in men are relatively asymptomatic and of low morbidity; the major consequence of infection in the male is the risk of transmission to a female partner. In women, gonococcal and chlamydial infections can result in PID, chronic abdominal and

The Reproductive System at a Glance, Fourth Edition. Linda J. Heffner and Danny J. Schust.

100 © 2014 John Wiley & Sons, Ltd. Published 2014 by John Wiley & Sons, Ltd. Companion Website: www.ataglanceseries.com/reproduction

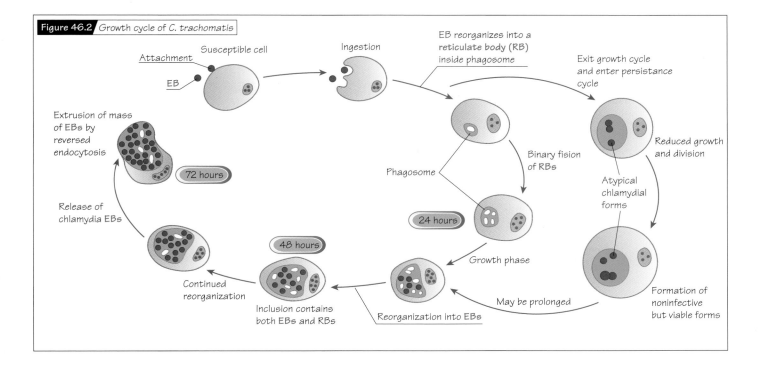

Figure 46.2 Growth cycle of C. trachomatis

Attachment — Susceptible cell

EB

Ingestion

EB reorganizes into a reticulate body (RB) inside phagosome

Exit growth cycle and enter persistence cycle

Reduced growth and division

Binary fision of RBs

Phagosome

Atypical chlamydial forms

Extrusion of mass of EBs by reversed endocytosis

72 hours

24 hours

Release of chlamydia EBs

48 hours

Growth phase

Formation of noninfective but viable forms

Continued reorganization

Inclusion contains both EBs and RBs

Reorganization into EBs

May be prolonged

pelvic pain, infertility and ectopic pregnancy. There is risk to the newborn infant from a birth canal infected with gonococci or chlamydiae. The greatest clinical difference between female infection with gonococci and CT is that **chlamydial PID is often asymptomatic. Hence, chlamydial infection is a major public health hazard because of the potential for undetected serious damage to the upper reproductive tracts of women**.

Chlamydia trachomatis is *the* most common STD in the USA and Europe. Chlamydiae are unique bacteria. Like viruses, they are obligate intracellular parasites and can only be propagated in cell culture. Chlamydia causes about 50% of the cases of nongonococcal urethritis in men. In women, chlamydia can cause mucopurulent cervicitis and the "urethral syndrome." In the latter, pain on urination is associated with the presence of white blood cells, but no bacteria, in the urine. Unlike gonorrhea, chlamydial infection of the upper genital tract often invades the endometrium and even the fallopian tubes without causing overt signs of PID. Such subclinical infection may first be recognized with diagnosis of the consequent infertility or ectopic pregnancy.

Several strains of chlamydia cause a unique disorder known as **lymphogranuloma venereum (LGV)**, a chronic disease that, like syphilis, has three clinical stages. The primary lesion of LGV is a small, inconspicuous papule of the genitalia that quickly and quietly disappears. The secondary stage of LGV is characterized by fever, malaise and either acute lymphadenitis of the inguinal region (bubo formation = inguinal syndrome) and/or acute hemorrhagic proctitis (anogenitorectal syndrome). Most people recover uneventfully from the second stage. In an unfortunate few, the chlamydiae persist in the anogenital tissues and incite a chronic inflammatory response that can cause genital tract ulcers, fistulae and strictures. LGV is endemic in much of the less developed world but sporadic in the USA and Europe. Neonates exposed to chlamydia in the birth canal may develop afebrile pneumonia or conjunctivitis that can progress to blindness.

Unlike gonococci, chlamydiae require prolonged treatment to eradicate the intracellular reservoir of the bacteria. First-line therapy is presently azithromycin or doxycycline. *In vitro* data and clinical experience indicate that *CT* may persist within certain infected cells for many years. Because of frequent coexistence of gonorrhea and chlamydial infection, most treatment regimens include antibiotics active against gonococci and chlamydia. True antibiotic resistance is rare in chlamydial infections.

Epidemiology of chlamydial infection
Chlamydia infection is a disease of the young. Additional risk factors include low socioeconomic status, a high number of sexual partners and oral contraceptive use. Barrier methods of contraception (condom, diaphragm, diaphragm plus spermicide) reduce risk.

Biology of chlamydia
The chlamydiae are structurally complex microorganisms. Like viruses, chlamydiae are obligate intracellular parasites. They are classified as bacteria because they contain both DNA and RNA. Like Gram-negative bacteria, they possess outer membrane proteins and an LPS. Chlamydiae differ from all other bacteria in that their growth cycle is characterized by transformation between two distinct forms: the **elementary body** and the **reticulate body** (Fig. 46.2). The elementary body is a highly infectious, rigid extracellular growth form that is metabolically inactive. The elementary body attaches to nonciliated columnar or cuboidal epithelial cells and induces ingestion by the host cell. The elementary body-containing phagosome does not fuse with host cell lysosomes, a characteristic crucial to CT survival and unique to only a few organisms (*Mycobacterium tuberculosis* is another). Within the phagosome, the elementary body reorganizes into a larger, metabolically active, fragile and noninfectious reticulate body. The reticulate bodies divide repeatedly by binary fission within the phagosome of the host cell. They will ultimately reorganize back into infectious elementary bodies that are released when the host cell dies.

There are 15 different serotypes or serovars of chlamydiae. These serovars are identified as A–K, Ba, and L_1, L_2 and L_3. Strains D–K are associated with chlamydial STDs. L_1, L_2 and L_3 cause LGV.

Figure 47.1 Life cycle of human papillomavirus

HPV

1. Infection of basal cells (E1/E2)
2. Integration of viral DNA (E1/E2 and E6/E7)
3. Viral DNA replication in squamous cells (E6/E7)
4. Viral assembly (L1/L2)
5. Shedding of HPV

Human papillomavirus

Infection with the **human papillomavirus (HPV) is the most common sexually transmitted infection (STI)** in the world. HPV is a wily pathogen that causes a spectrum of clinical diseases, all of which involve cutaneous or mucosal squamous surfaces. From the evolutionary standpoint, HPVs are very successful infectious agents because they induce chronic infections that have no systemic sequelae and rarely kill the host. Instead they periodically shed large amounts of infectious virus for transmission to naïve individuals.

The broad spectrum of genital HPV infection includes: (i) latent infection; (ii) clinically apparent lesions (condylomata acuminata, warts); and (iii) HPV-associated neoplasia. Latent infections are identified by the presence of HPV DNA in tissue samples acquired for epidemiologic study. In the absence of tissue collection, latent infections would go unrecognized because neither microscopic nor visible lesions are present. Overt **genital warts, also known as condyloma acuminata**, are flesh-colored, pink or pigmented papules with a frond-like surface. Sessile warts, or flat condyloma-like lesions, are less common, accounting for only 20% of visible genital warts. Most genital warts in men are on the penis. In women, they are found most often at the vaginal introitus and on the labia. Most genital warts are asymptomatic. When symptoms do occur, they are often secondary to local friction-induced irritation from clothing or intercourse. **HPV-associated neoplasias include intraepithelial lesions of the cervix (CIN) and vulva (VIN) and invasive carcinomas at both sites**. Cervical cancer is discussed in detail in Chapter 44.

Because most genital warts are sexually transmitted, their presence indicates risk for other STIs. Treatment of genital warts involves cryotherapy or topical application of agents that cause cytolysis.

Epidemiology of HPV

The primary risk factor for HPV infection is sexual activity. It is estimated that 75% of sexually active women will acquire latent HPV infection. Fortunately, most HPV infections are transient; up to 90% of infections in women will resolve spontaneously within 2 years of acquisition. Unfortunately, persistent infection is more common with HPV genotypes that have neoplastic potential.

Although rare, it is possible to acquire HPV through nonsexual transmission. Neonates can become infected during delivery.

Biology of human papillomaviruses

HPV is a member of the Papovaviridae family of DNA viruses. Other well-known members of this family are the polyomaviruses (polio virus and SV40). Of the 130 different HPV genotypes identified to date, about 40 are associated with genital lesions. Types 6 and 11 are most commonly identified in genital warts, and types 16 and 18 are most closely associated with neoplasia (high-risk subtypes). HPV subtypes 1–5 are associated with common skin warts and plantar warts.

The success of HPV as an infectious agent is directly linked to a virus replication cycle that effectively evades immunologic detection by the host. The virus infects primitive keratinocytes in the basal layers of squamous epithelia followed by a round of viral DNA replication that appears independent of the host cell cycle (Fig. 47.1). Once the infected keratinocyte enters the proliferative compartment of the epithelium, viral gene expression is minimal. The oncogenes $E6$ and $E7$ are highly repressed by the viral genes $E1$ and $E2$ until the infected keratinocyte exits the cell cycle and enters the uppermost differentiating compartment (Table 47.1). Thus, high levels of viral protein synthesis and assembly only occur in the upper layers of the squamous epithelium. In this infectious cycle, the virus hitches a ride in the keratinocyte at the beginning of its journey and replicates in cells that will terminally differentiate and die by natural causes. Thus, there is no viral-induced cytolysis, necrosis or inflammation. Because there is no blood-borne phase of the HPV life cycle and only minimal amounts of replicating virus are exposed to immune defense, the virus is essentially invisible to the host. It is only when host integration occurs with $E1$ and $E2$ disruption, that $E6$ and $E7$ are overexpressed. $E6$ and $E7$ are capable of interfering with important tumor suppressor proteins in the host cell. Their overexpression is associated with neoplastic transformation, explaining the oncogenic potential of HPV.

HPV vaccines are effective because they circumvent the viral epithelial evasion strategies by introducing virus antigens through an intramuscular route. An immune cascade resulting in a robust T-cell-dependent B-cell response generates high levels of $L1$ specific neutralizing antibodies and immune memory.

The Reproductive System at a Glance, Fourth Edition. Linda J. Heffner and Danny J. Schust.
102

Table 47.1 Important human papillomavirus (HPV) genes

E1*	Necessary for viral DNA replication
	May have a role as a repressor of immortalization
E2*	Necessary for viral DNA replication along with E1
E6†	Interacts with p53; transforming signal
E7†	Interacts with Rb-1; strong transforming signal
L1	Major capsid protein
L2	Minor capsid protein

* Mutations in E1 and/or E2 result in integration of viral DNA into host DNA.
† Disruption of growth regulation necessary to propagate virus.

Herpes simplex virus

Genital herpes is an STD that does not go away. Instead, the responsible agent, **herpes simplex virus (HSV)**, establishes latent genital infection in the sacral dorsal root ganglia. It can be reactivated from latency by fever, sun exposure and hormonal changes. Herpetic infection causes the greatest morbidity in the neonate, who acquires it from the genital tract of the mother at delivery, and in immunocompromised patients for whom its disseminated form can be life-threatening.

There are two distinct serological types of HSV: HSV-1 and HSV-2. HSV-1 infection is typically asymptomatic and nearly ubiquitous. It is transmitted by primary infection of the respiratory tract. HSV-1 has been found in the trigeminal ganglion of 80% of cadavers.

HSV-2 has a predilection for genital disease, although HSV-1 infections of the genitalia and HSV-2 infections of the oral cavity do occur. HSV-2 is much more likely than HSV-1 to become a latent infection of the sacral ganglion and to cause neonatal disease.

Patients with herpetic infections present with three clinical scenarios: **primary first episode**, **nonprimary first episode** and **recurrent episodes**. These presentations inform our understanding of the biology and epidemiology of genital HSV infections. First episodes describe the initial recognition by the patient or health-care provider that a genital herpes infection is occurring. In primary first episodes, no HSV antibodies can be detected in acute phase serum samples, demonstrating that there has been no prior HSV infection. HSV antibodies will be present at the time of the first recognized genital herpes outbreak in nonprimary first episodes. Recurrent episodes require recognition that the patient has had a prior episode(s) of symptomatic HSV. The severity of clinical manifestations and the incidence of complications at presentation vary according to whether the infection is primary, nonprimary or recurrent.

Primary genital HSV disease is typically the most severe although it can be totally asymptomatic. Over 80% of patients with primary genital HSV will have local painful penile or vulvar lesions, dysuria, urethral or vaginal discharge and painful inguinal adenopathy. The mean duration of viral shedding from mucocutaneous lesions in primary genital HSV-2 infections is 2–3 weeks. Nonprimary first infections tend to be milder than primary first infections, presumably because acquired humoral and cellular immunity partially contain infectious spread.

Recurrent genital HSV-2 disease typically involves painful recrudescence of the mucocutaneous lesions on the penis or vulva and cervix. Local viral shedding occurs at the site of lesions, although cervical shedding has also been documented in the absence of visible cervical lesions. Systemic symptoms are absent. The mean duration of symptoms and viral shedding is much shorter with recurrences.

Medications that inhibit viral DNA synthesis have been developed to treat the symptoms of HSV infection. Treatment will stop viral DNA replication and spread but will neither prevent latent infections nor eradicate the virus.

Abstinence from sexual contact with an infected partner when lesions are visible is the only way to prevent genital HSV infection. Unfortunately, even this is not completely protective because transmission can occur during asymptomatic viral shedding. Condoms are also not completely protective. The penile shaft may be partially exposed to the vulva during intercourse using a condom. In addition, HSV is capable of penetrating latex.

Epidemiology of genital HSV infection

Symptomatic genital HSV infection accounts for 2–4% of visits to STD clinics in the UK and the USA. Genital HSV infections are reported more commonly among Caucasians than non-Caucasians. A higher prevalence of anti-HSV antibodies is noted with decreasing age at first coitus and with increasing number of sexual partners.

The incidence of neonatal herpes is about 1 in 7500 live births.

Biology of HSV

HSV is a member of the herpesvirus class of DNA viruses. Herpesviridae include the two serotypes of HSV, cytomegalovirus (CMV), varicella zoster (chickenpox, shingles) and Epstein–Barr virus (mononucleosis, chronic fatigue syndrome). Herpesviruses would be better called "complex" rather than "simplex" because they have the most complicated structure and replication cycles of all the viruses.

Genital HSV is acquired by sexual contact with contaminated secretions or lesions. Herpesviruses are very susceptible to desiccation and extremes of temperature, making transmission by fomites very rare. Once the virus has gained access to mucosal cells, it destroys the host DNA during productive replication of its own and kills the cell. HSV spreads by contiguity to adjacent cells and tracks toward autonomic nerve endings. Mucosal and skin cells infected with HSV produce serous transudates that result in the classic vesicles seen in the disorder.

Following primary genital mucocutaneous infection, HSV virions travel to the dorsal root ganglia of the sacral plexus (S_2–S_4) via the intra-axonal route. Here, they persist in a nonreplicative state until reactivation. Reactivation is heralded by a dramatic increase in viral DNA synthesis. This is followed by spread of virus back down the sensory neurons to the skin.

HSV in pregnancy and the neonate

Ninety per cent of women with primary genital HSV-2 infection shed virus from their cervix during the acute infection. This level drops to 70% both in women with primary genital HSV-1 infection and in women with nonprimary first episodes of genital HSV-2 infection. These numbers stand in stark contrast to the 12–20% rate of cervical shedding among women with recurrent external genital lesions. Therefore, it is not surprising that 50% of pregnant women with primary genital HSV will transmit infection to the neonate while only 5% of women with recurrent genital HSV will do so. Neonatal herpetic infections are life-threatening. They may be prevented with appropriate use of cesarean delivery.

48 The special cases of syphilis and human immunodeficiency virus

Syphilis

Natural history of untreated syphilis

Syphilis is caused by the spirochete bacterium, *Treponema pallidum*, which enters the body through miniscule breaks in the skin of the external genitalia that occur during sexual intercourse. Once the spirochete has entered, the untreated disease progresses through **four consecutive stages: primary, secondary, latent and tertiary syphilis**. Antibiotic treatment at any stage short of tertiary can prevent the late, life-threatening sequelae of the disease. Syphilis may also be transmitted from a woman to her fetus at any point during pregnancy, with serious consequences.

The primary lesion of syphilis, the **chancre**, develops in venereal locations close to where *T. pallidum* typically enters the body: the penis, labia, perineum, anus or rectum. Chancres are painless, small papules that persist for 1–2 months and heal spontaneously.

The secondary stage of syphilis is a disseminated form. Blood-borne spirochetes populate the dermis throughout the body causing a widespread papular rash over the trunk and extremities. Because the disease is systemic, fever, myalgias, lymphadenopathy, sore throat and headache are common. Secondary syphilis can also be associated with immune complex deposition in the joints, kidneys and eyes, leading to arthritis, glomerulonephritis, nephrotic syndrome and uveitis. Untreated secondary syphilis resolves over 4–12 weeks, leaving the patient symptom free. The subsequent months to years until the onset of symptoms of tertiary syphilis is known as the latent period.

Tertiary syphilis usually appears many years after the disseminated stage. Tertiary syphilis can involve multiple organs, including the cardiovascular and nervous systems. Overall, about one-quarter of untreated patients develop recognizable late (tertiary) complications of syphilis, one-quarter have asymptomatic lesions demonstrable at autopsy and half have no anatomic lesions attributable to syphilis present at autopsy. About half of the patients with symptomatic tertiary syphilis will die as a direct result of the disease, typically of cardiovascular complications.

Infection of the placenta and fetus will occur in virtually 100% of pregnant women who suffer the spirochetemia accompanying primary or secondary syphilis. Complications of syphilis in pregnancy include miscarriage, stillbirth, premature delivery and congenital syphilis. The manifestations of congenital syphilis are protean. Its neonatal mortality rate is 50%.

Syphilis is treated with penicillin in all but highly allergic patients.

Epidemiology of syphilis

Syphilis was very common in many parts of the world until antibiotic therapy became available in the 1940s. The prevalence of the disease fell dramatically after World War II but began to increase again in the 1960s. Up to 75% of cases go unreported. Women and men at high risk for contracting syphilis are young, from lower socioeconomic groups, and have multiple sexual partners. Some 10–50 syphilitic organisms are sufficient to cause infection and about one-third of the sexual contacts of an infected person will become infected. The incidence of congenital syphilis parallels that in women and is increasing. Mandatory prenatal screening has reduced the incidence of late congenital syphilis; late or absent prenatal care is the biggest risk factor for congenital syphilis.

Biology of *T. pallidum*

Treponema pallidum is a member of the bacterial order *Spirochaetaceae*, and closely related to two other treponemas responsible for human disease: *Treponema pertenue*, which causes yaws, and *T. carateum*, which causes pinta. Neither electron microscopic examination nor DNA analyses can distinguish between these three organisms. It is believed that the different diseases that develop reflect adaptations of the organism and the host to different points of entry into the body.

Treponema pallidum is a relatively fragile organism that cannot survive for more than a few hours outside moist areas of the body. Its microbiology is very poorly understood because the organism cannot be maintained in cell culture.

Most of the manifestations of syphilis are secondary to the inflammatory reaction caused by the organism. Polymorphonuclear cells arriving at the site of the inoculum ingest the spirochetes but do not kill them. Lymphocytes and macrophages are recruited to the site. They also surround, but do not kill the treponemes. Antitreponemal antibodies are produced, sometimes in quantities that cause immune complex glomerulonephritis. It remains both amazing and unknown how *T. pallidum* is able to evade host defenses and establish an infection. The site of primary infection is surrounded by a mucoid material composed of hyaluronic acid and chondroitin sulfate that may alter the host defenses. The best clue available to explain the persistence of disease is the finding that delayed type sensitivity to treponemal antigens is absent in secondary syphilis. New spirochetes inoculated into the system are not infectious while the original infection persists. This is a common mechanism in chronic parasitic diseases, called "premunition"; the host resists reinfection but cannot clear the initial infection.

Once the systemic phase of the infection is established, spirochetes are present virtually everywhere in the infected tissues. However, inflammation occurs preferentially around small vessels and causes intimal hyperplasia and obliterative endarteritis. The subsequent focal ischemic necrosis and fibrosis are responsible for the many late manifestations of the disease.

The inflammatory changes caused by the spirochetes are most striking in congenital syphilis. The placenta is diffusely fibrotic with inflammation and necrosis of the fetal blood vessels in the placental villi. The resulting vascular insufficiency leads to poor fetal growth (**intrauterine growth restriction**) and **stillbirth**. Fibrosis of the liver and spleen cause fetal anemia. Compensatory extramedullary hematopoiesis promotes hepatosplenomegaly and the development of pleural effusions and ascites (**fetal hydrops**). Some infants will have a skin rash that closely resembles that of secondary syphilis. A runny nasal discharge loaded with spirochetes (**snuffles**) may be the only hint of congenital syphilis at birth.

The late manifestations of syphilis, both congenital and tertiary, involve vasculitis and parenchymal damage in the central nervous system.

Human immunodeficiency virus

Natural history of untreated HIV infections

The first description of human disease associated with HIV infection surfaced in the early 1980s. Acute infection was reported to cause a "mononucleosis-like syndrome" with fever, malaise, muscle aches, headache, fatigue, generalized rash, sore throat, lymphadenopathy and characteristic mucocutaneous lesions. The rapidity of symptom onset

The Reproductive System at a Glance, Fourth Edition. Linda J. Heffner and Danny J. Schust.

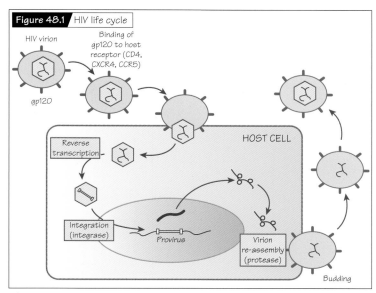

Figure 48.1 HIV life cycle

HIV virion

Binding of gp120 to host receptor (CD4, CXCR4, CCR5)

gp120

HOST CELL

Reverse transcription

Integration (integrase)

Provirus

Virion re-assembly (protease)

Budding

after initial contact may reflect the route of viral entry and the viral load of the exposure. Symptoms of primary infection often persist for 2–3 weeks before resolving spontaneously. The disease then enters an asymptomatic phase. This can last from several months to many years. The length of this symptom-free phase appears to depend on the pathogenicity of the infecting viral strain. Coinfection with other viruses or other sexually transmitted disease (STD) pathogens may speed disease progression. During the asymptomatic phase, viral replication continues within infected lymphoid cells (mainly CD4+ T cells). Infected immune cells are destroyed by the virus and, eventually, the host becomes immunocompromised. In this immunocompromised state, the HIV-infected individual is vulnerable to a variety of opportunistic viral, bacterial, fungal and parasitic infections. Opportunistic pathogens such as *Pneumocystis carinii*, *Cryptosporidium* and *Cryptococcus* seldom affect individuals with normally functioning immune systems but can be deadly in those infected with HIV. Patients who are severely immunocompromised are also at risk for the development of certain neoplasms, including Kaposi sarcoma, human papillomavirus-related cervical cancers and some lymphomas. The development of opportunistic infections or neoplasms in a patient infected with HIV defines the acute immunodeficiency syndrome (AIDS). Patient who die of AIDS typically succumb to complications of an opportunistic infection or neoplasm.

Epidemiology of HIV infections

HIV has infected over 60 million people worldwide, and 35 million are presently living with the disease. The developing world accounts for 95% of infections, with over 25 million of those presently infected living in sub-Saharan Africa. The most important risk factor for acquiring HIV infection and succumbing to its complications is poverty.

Viral transmission occurs through direct contact with bodily fluids, most often semen or blood. Viral spread can occur via sexual contact, via parenteral exposure (intravenous drug abuse and transfusions) or via perinatal transmission. The latter can occur during pregnancy (transmission across the placenta), at delivery or during breastfeeding. Only 25% of children born to untreated HIV-positive mothers will acquire the infection, although this rate can be decreased to less than 1–2% with aggressive antenatal and perinatal therapy. Over 90% of HIV infections occur via heterosexual transmission. HIV is more readily transmitted from the male to female (1 in 500–1000 acts of receptive vaginal intercourse) than female to male (1 in 2000–2500 acts of insertive vaginal intercourse).

Biology of HIV

HIV is a retrovirus. Its genetic material is carried as RNA wrapped in a viral protein coating. The viral surface expresses a receptor called gp120 that binds specifically to receptors on lymphoid cells (Fig. 48.1). Binding promotes viral entry into host cells. Host receptors and co-receptors for viral entry include CCR5, a chemokine receptor on macrophages, CXCR4, a chemokine receptor expressed on T cells, and CD4, a marker for T helper cells that is also expressed on macrophages and dendritic cells. Once viral entry has occurred, infected cells will fuse with CD4+ T helper cells. Viral propagation will continue largely in CD4+ cells.

After entry into a host cell, the retrovirus uses reverse transcriptase to make a DNA copy of its viral RNA genome. The virus then uses an enzyme called integrase to insert its newly synthesized DNA into the host genome and the host cell machinery makes multiple copies of the HIV genome. The virus finally employs an enzyme called protease to reassemble the viral envelope. Viral particles then exit the host cell via budding to infect surrounding receptor-laden immune cells. Multiple viral progeny will be produced within a single infected host cell before it expires.

Reverse transcriptase (RT), integrase and protease are virus-specific enzymes. They can therefore serve as targets for directed therapeutic interventions. Over 20 FDA-approved medications are now available to treat HIV infections. None are curative and optimal therapies typically use combinations of two to four medications. Available antiretroviral medications inhibit each of the HIV-specific enzymes: the HIV protease (protease inhibitors), the RT enzyme [nucleoside RT inhibitors (NRTI), non-nucleoside RT inhibitors (NNRTI)], and HIV integrase (integrase inhibitors). Inhibitors of HIV viral entry have recently been released.

In developed countries, careful therapeutic interventions, combined with close monitoring of CD4+ T-cell counts and viral loads, have radically improved the prognosis for those infected with HIV. Further advances are challenged by the fact that the HIV reverse transcriptase enzyme makes many mistakes during replication of the viral genome. The virus has no way to readily correct these mistakes. This allows for rapid viral mutation and, unfortunately, the development of resistance to antiretroviral medications. In underdeveloped countries, where the prevalence of disease is highest, medications are scarce or completely unavailable.

Index

Page numbers in *italic* denote figures, those in **bold** denote tables.

The at a Glance series

Popular double-page spread format • Coverage of core knowledge
Full-colour throughout • Self-assessment to test your knowledge • Expert authors

www.wileymedicaleducation.com

WILEY-
BLACKWELL

The Lecture Notes series

The *Lecture Notes* series provides concise, yet thorough, introductions to core areas of the undergraduate curriculum, covering both the basic science and the clinical approaches that all medical students and junior doctors need to know.

www.lecturenoteseries.com
www.wileymedicaleducation.com

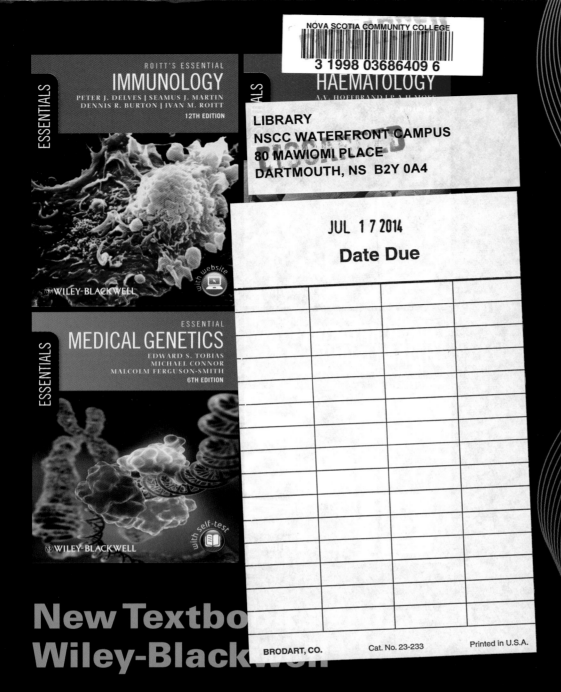
New Textbo
Wiley-Blackwell

All written by renowned names in their fields, they feature fully updated and new artwork, MCQs and answers for self-assessment, and an enhanced Wiley Desktop Edition as standard - FREE upon purchase of the book. This provides an interactive digital version of the book featuring downloadable text and images, highlighting and note taking facilities, book-marking, cross-referencing, in-text searching, and linking to references and glossary terms.

www.wileymedicaleducation.com
www.wiley.com/go/essentialsseries

10-24646